Regenerative Medicine: A Guide to Stem Cell Therapy

Revolutionizing Medicine, Restoring Hope, and Embracing the Future of Healing

S. B. Wade

© Copyright 2024, Sandra Waite - All rights reserved.

The content contained within this book may not be reproduced, duplicated or transmitted without direct written permission from the author or the publisher.

Under no circumstances will any blame or legal responsibility be held against the publisher, or author, for any damages, reparation, or monetary loss due to the information contained within this book, either directly or indirectly.

Legal Notice:

This book is copyright protected. It is only for personal use. You cannot amend, distribute, sell, use, quote or paraphrase any part, or the content within this book, without the consent of the author or publisher.

Disclaimer Notice:

Please note the information contained within this document is for educational and entertainment purposes only. All effort has been executed to present accurate, up to date, reliable, complete information. No warranties of any kind are declared or implied. Readers acknowledge that the author is not engaged in the rendering of legal, financial, medical or professional advice. The content within this book has been derived from various sources. Please consult a licensed professional before attempting any techniques outlined in this book.

By reading this document, the reader agrees that under no circumstances is the author responsible for any losses, direct or indirect, that are incurred as a result of the use of the information contained within this document, including, but not limited to, errors, omissions, or inaccuracies.

Table of Contents

INTRODUCTION 1

CHAPTER 1: THE SCIENCE OF STEM CELLS...5

    INTRODUCTION TO STEM CELLS 5
        The Cell Cycle...7
        Telomeres and Their Significance..7
        Cell Senescence and Its Implications...7
    THE UNIQUE QUALITIES OF STEM CELLS 8
    ADVANCEMENTS IN IMAGING AND MONITORING STEM CELLS 9
    STEM CELL NICHES AND MICROENVIRONMENTS 10
    REGENERATION POTENTIAL..11
    GENETIC AND EPIGENETIC REGULATION IN STEM CELLS 13
        Genetic Influence on Pluripotency and Differentiation.................13
        Epigenetic Marks and Their Influence...14
        Manipulating Epigenetic Modifications..14
    HISTORY OF STEM CELL RESEARCH 16
        Technical Advances in Stem Cell Isolation and Cultivation............18
    STEM CELL MARKERS AND IDENTIFICATION 19

CHAPTER 2: STEM CELL THERAPY INDICATIONS 23

    INTRODUCTION 23
    SUCCESS STORIES...23
    GENERALIZED CONDITIONS TREATED WITH STEM CELL THERAPY 24
    TREATING NEUROLOGICAL DISORDERS WITH STEM CELL THERAPY 25
        Parkinson's Disease..25
        Alzheimer's Disease..25
        Spinal Cord Injuries...26
    STEM CELL THERAPY IN ORTHOPEDICS 26
        Treating Joint Pain..27
        Osteoarthritis Management...27
        Cartilage Injuries and Repair..28
    AUTOIMMUNE DISEASES 28

Real-World Applications and Success Stories 29
Cardiac and Vascular Conditions 31
   Myocardial Infarction 31
   Peripheral Artery Disease (PAD) 32
Stem Cell Therapy in Other Conditions 33
   Diabetes 33
   Pulmonary Diseases 34
   Liver Disorders 36
   Cancer Treatment 36
Future Directions in Stem Cell Therapy 36
Revealing the Potential of Stem Cell Therapy 37
   Organ Regeneration 38
   Bioartificial Organs 38
   "De-Aging" Stem Cells and Life Extension 39
   Challenges and Ethical Considerations 40

CHAPTER 3: TYPES OF STEM CELL THERAPY 42

Autologous Stem Cell Therapy 42
   Understanding Autologous Stem Cell Therapy 42
   The Procedure 43
   Potential Benefits 44
   Treatments 45
Allogeneic Stem Cell Therapy 46
   The Procedure 46
   Applications 48
Induced Pluripotent Stem Cells (iPSCs) 49
   Creating iPSCs: A Breakthrough in Cellular Reprogramming 49
   Applications of iPSCs: Unleashing Regenerative Potential 50
Challenges Faced in Stem Cell Research 52

CHAPTER 4: EVALUATING STEM CELL THERAPY 54

The Promise and Perils of Regenerative Medicine 54
Serious Safety Concerns With Regenerative Medicine 54
The Path Ahead 55
Benefits and Potential Outcomes 56
   A Multitude of Conditions 56

Consider the account of a young girl, once bound by the limitations of cerebral palsy, who found a new lease on life through stem cell therapy. Her journey, documented by medical practitioners and celebrated by her family, speaks volumes of the strides she's made—from tentative steps to a confident walk, from fragmented speech to clear articulation. Yet, alongside her success, we are reminded by her doctors of the road still ahead, the research still required, and the careful consideration that must be given to each case.

In the annals of Reddit—a repository of raw, unfiltered experiences—individuals with amyotrophic lateral sclerosis (ALS) share their encounters with stem cell therapy. One recounts the tempered hope that blossomed with treatment, a gentle improvement in their condition where once there was only decline. Though far from a cure, these small victories represent monumental triumphs for those grappling with the relentless progression of ALS.

It's important to weave these threads of hope with the strands of reality. For every story of improvement, there are reminders of the therapy's developing state—successes are not universal, and the science is still unfolding. Every testimonial is hopeful, yet each is tempered in the gentle warning that stem cell therapy is not a universal cure, but a potential path to betterment that must be walked with caution and clear-eyed understanding.

The path to understanding stem cell therapy is fraught with dense scientific terminology and complex concepts. This book demystifies the subject, clearing the fog. It is intended as a comprehensive yet accessible guide that unravels the intricacies of this groundbreaking field.

By the end of *Regenerative Medicine,* you will not simply hold a collection of success stories or cautionary tales; you will possess a map through the complex topography of stem cell therapy.

This book is designed to transform information into action, uncertainty into understanding, and passivity into empowerment.

You will emerge with a vivid picture of:

- The sheer breadth of stem cell therapy's reach, touching lives affected by diverse conditions.

- The depth of knowledge required to discerningly consider these treatments, understanding the scientific principles that govern them.

- The height of ethical considerations that accompany such profound medical interventions, ensuring respect for the sanctity of life and individual choice.

Here is what you can expect from each chapter:

- Chapter 1: "The Science of Stem Cells" introduces you to stem cells, laying the groundwork for understanding their regenerative capabilities.

- Chapter 2: "The Science of Healing" explores how stem cells are used to repair damaged tissue and what that means for medical treatments.

- Chapter 3: "Successes and Setbacks" provides a balanced look at the real-world impact of stem cell therapies, including the limitations and challenges.

- Chapter 4: "Stem Cell Evaluation" explores the benefits, safety considerations, clinical trials, regulations, and legalities are outlined.

- Chapter 5: "The Decision-Making Process" guides you in making informed decisions about stem cell therapy.

- Chapter 6: "Maximizing the Benefits of Stem Cell Therapy" unlocks the full potential of stem cell therapy.

- Chapter 7: "Challenges in Stem Cell Therapy" outlines the obstacles and hurdles that researchers, clinicians, patients, and society face as stem cell therapy becomes more widely accepted.

- Chapter 8: "Ethical Considerations and Future Perspectives" explores the ethical dilemmas shaping both practice and research in stem cell therapy, and considers the guiding principles for practitioners and researchers.

With each chapter, you will find yourself better equipped to manage the future of healing that stem cell therapy presents. Whether you are a patient, a caregiver, or simply someone fascinated by the prospects of medical science, this guide is for you.

Chapter 1:
The Science of Stem Cells

Introduction to Stem Cells

Imagine a single cell, no larger than a grain of salt, with the monumental potential to regenerate, repair, and replenish any type of tissue in the human body. This is not the premise of a futuristic novel; this is the reality of stem cells. Did you know that stem cells can be trained to mimic the functions of other cells, so much so that they could potentially repair a damaged heart, restore vision, or even reverse the effects of neurodegenerative diseases? They are the body's raw materials, the builders and healers within us, poised to transform medicine as we know it.

As we stand on the cusp of medical innovation, these microscopic marvels are leading the charge, offering us a glimpse into a future where the word "incurable" becomes obsolete. In this chapter, we unravel the mysteries of stem cells, exploring their remarkable regenerative capabilities, and how they are steering us towards a new horizon in medicine. Prepare to delve into the world of these cellular powerhouses and understand why their discovery is hailed as one of the greatest advancements in modern science.

Stem cells are full of potential—they are unspecialized cells with the ability to become any of the cells that make up our organs and tissues. They are the chameleons of the cellular world, with two defining powers. First, they possess the remarkable capability for self-renewal, meaning they can divide and replicate themselves for long periods. Second, they can differentiate, which is a scientific way of saying they can transform into specialized cells, whether it be a neuron in the brain, a red blood cell carrying oxygen through our veins, or a cardiomyocyte making our hearts beat.

The main types are

- Embryonic stem cells are exactly what they sound like: tissue collected from embryos, and are pluripotent—they can become almost any cell of the body. Their incredible versatility makes them both powerful and controversial.

- Adult stem cells are more like seasoned professionals. Located in tissues like the bone marrow, brain, and liver, they typically generate cells only within their own tissue type, a property known as multipotency. These are the most well-known, because of their use in bone marrow transplant.

- The pluripotent stem cells (iPSCs) are the third type. Scientists call them the shapeshifters of the stem cell universe. These cells can be reprogrammed to a state that allows them to change into almost any cell. This revolutionary technique means cells from your own body could one day be used to repair your tissues, offering personalized medicine without the ethical concerns of embryonic stem cells.

Each type of stem cell comes with unique characteristics and possibilities, as well as challenges and limitations. Understanding these allows us not only to marvel at their capabilities but also to manage the complex ethical, medical, and research settings they inhabit.

The Cell Cycle

All cells cycle in growth and reproduction. This cycle can be distilled into several distinct phases: interphase (comprising G1, S, and G2 phases) and mitosis. The cell grows, its DNA duplicates, then organizes. Next, mitosis occurs and the cell becomes two genetically identical cells.

This regulated cycle is essential for the maintenance, repair, and replenishment of tissues and organs within the body. However, for most cells, the cycle is finite. Over time, as cells divide repeatedly, their ability to replicate becomes compromised due to a phenomenon known as telomere shortening.

Telomeres and Their Significance

Telomeres are like the protective caps on the ends of shoelaces, safeguarding our DNA from fraying or degradation during replication. They consist of repetitive sequences of nucleotides and serve as a buffer, ensuring that vital genetic information remains intact during cell division. Each time a cell divides, its telomeres shorten, acting as a sort of cellular clock that ticks down with each replication.

Cell Senescence and Its Implications

As the telomeres shorten with subsequent divisions, the telomeres become critically short. This signals the cell to enter a state known as senescence or cellular aging. The cell can no longer divide and aid in tissue regeneration. Instead, it may secrete inflammatory signals that can have detrimental effects on surrounding cells and tissues.

The Unique Qualities of Stem Cells

Now, let's consider how stem cells fit into this intricate puzzle. Stem cells, by their very nature, possess a remarkable ability to defy the limits of the cell cycle. Unlike most cells in our bodies, they can self-renew and divide while maintaining the integrity of their telomeres. This intrinsic quality sets them apart as the true champions of tissue regeneration and repair.

Stem cells also exhibit another exceptional attribute called pluripotency or multipotency. These cells carry the ability to become multiple cell types in the body. Multipotent stem cells, which are commonly located in adult tissues, exhibit the ability to transform into a restricted set of cell types, highly prized for their role in tissue-specific restoration.

Stem cells, with their extended telomeres and ability to bypass the inevitability of senescence, stand as a beacon of hope in the quest for regenerative medicine. They offer the promise of replenishing damaged or aging tissues, mitigating the limitations imposed by telomere shortening and cellular aging in other cell types.

The cell cycle, telomeres, and cell senescence are critical factors governing the life and functionality of our cells. Stem cells, with their unique ability to circumvent the limitations imposed by telomere shortening and senescence, hold the key to unlocking the potential of regenerative medicine. They represent a remarkable exception in the cellular world, offering the possibility of rejuvenating and healing our bodies, making them an invaluable asset in the realm of medical research and treatment.

Advancements in Imaging and Monitoring Stem Cells

High-resolution live-cell imaging is a recent development. This technique allows scientists to observe stem cells in real-time without disrupting their surroundings. By using specialized microscopes and fluorescent markers, researchers can track the movements, division, and interactions of stem cells within tissues. This capability has shed light on the intricate processes involved in tissue regeneration and disease progression.

Additionally, the emergence of non-invasive imaging modalities, such as magnetic resonance imaging (MRI) and positron emission tomography (PET), has enabled the tracking of stem cells in vivo, within living organisms. These techniques have proven invaluable in monitoring the fate and distribution of transplanted stem cells, opening new possibilities for regenerative medicine and cell-based therapies.

Computational biology plays a crucial role in modeling stem cell behavior and predicting their differentiation pathways. With the help of powerful computer simulations and mathematical models, scientists can analyze large datasets generated from experiments and make predictions about how stem cells respond to various stimuli. This approach has been instrumental in identifying key factors that influence stem cell fate, helping researchers design more effective strategies for tissue regeneration and disease treatment.

Advancements in imaging technologies and the integration of computational biology have revolutionized our ability to study stem cells. These tools provide a window into the complex world of stem cell biology, enabling us to understand their behavior in unprecedented detail and harness their potential for medical applications.

Stem Cell Niches and Microenvironments

Stem cell niches are the environments in which stem cells live. These niches play a critical role in regulating the self-renewal and differentiation of stem cells. Regenerative medicine requires understanding of the niches to utilize stem cells.

The niches reside in tissues and organs, creating ecosystems that sustain and maintain the stem cells. Within these niches, stem cells receive signals from neighboring cells, extracellular matrix components, and soluble factors that dictate their fate. These signals can push stem cells to either self-renew, maintaining their stem cell identity, or differentiate into specialized cell types to contribute to tissue repair or growth.

Tissue engineering has emerged as a promising approach to replicate stem cell niches in vitro. Researchers are working to mimic the complex microenvironment of these niches in the lab, allowing for better control over stem cell behavior and fate. By designing synthetic scaffolds and culturing conditions that mimic the cues found in natural niches, scientists aim to create environments that enhance stem cell proliferation and differentiation for therapeutic purposes.

Understanding and replicating stem cell niches also have implications for cancer research. Tumor-initiating cells, often considered similar to stem cells, can hijack the cues from their niches to promote unchecked growth. Studying and targeting these niche interactions may offer novel strategies for cancer treatment.

Stem cell niches are pivotal in governing the behavior of stem cells. Replicating these microenvironments in vitro through tissue engineering is a promising avenue for controlling and directing stem cell fate, holding great potential for regenerative medicine and cancer therapies.

As we examine these concepts, we'll share stories that bring to life the incredible potential of stem cells. From the child whose life was changed by a bone marrow transplant to the breakthroughs in creating iPSCs that won the Nobel Prize, these narratives illustrate the real-world impact of the science we're exploring. With each account, stem cells will shift from abstract entities to powerful protagonists in the stories of healing and hope.

Regeneration Potential

The concept of regeneration has fascinated humanity for centuries, drawing images of mythological creatures that could heal instantly. In the realm of science, stem cells are our closest reality to this mythic regeneration. Their capability to repair and rejuvenate tissues is not just a dream of the future, but an unfolding reality of today's medicine.

Regenerative medicine refers to using stem cells to repair damaged tissues. Unlike most cells in our body, which serve specific functions, stem cells remain on standby, ready to be called into action. When damage occurs, signals from the affected area attract stem cells, prompting them to migrate to the site. Once there, these adaptable cells start to proliferate and differentiate into the types of cells needed for repair, be it muscle, bone, or neurons.

Let's look at heart disease, a condition in which the heart muscle cells sustain damage and lack the innate ability to self-repair. Scientists have harnessed stem cells to craft fresh heart muscle cells, subsequently introducing them into the patients' cardiac tissues. This innovative approach holds the promise of enhancing heart function and recovery. This is no small feat in the world of medicine where heart disease remains a leading cause of death.

Then there's the regenerative potential in neurology. Diseases like Parkinson's, which arise from the loss of specific neurons, are in the crosshairs of stem cell therapy. By growing new dopamine-producing cells from stem cells and implanting them into the brains of patients, there is potential to replace what has been lost to the disease.

The mechanisms by which stem cells are harnessed in regenerative medicine are intricate and require a delicate balance of conditions. It is a symphony of biological signals and responses that guide stem cells to behave in ways that benefit the host tissue. For instance, in stem cell therapy, cells are often cultured and manipulated in the lab to enhance their healing properties before being introduced to the patient's body.

Take, for instance, the story of a young athlete with a chronic knee injury, where traditional treatments offered little hope. Stem cell therapy provided a regenerative option where cells were injected into the injured area, stimulating repair and allowing her to return to sports.

These examples are not isolated miracles but represent a growing field of study. Success stories are increasingly common, yet they come with the caveat that stem cell therapy is not a universal cure. Researchers are diligently working to understand and improve the mechanisms behind these treatments, ensuring safety and efficacy.

Stem cells are lifelines of hope, avenues to a future where the body's own cells could offer the most personalized and effective treatments. We'll explore these topics with a sense of grounded optimism, aware of the current limitations but eager for the possibilities that lie just over the horizon of current science.

Genetic and Epigenetic Regulation in Stem Cells

Understanding genetic and epigenetic factors within stem cells is central to unraveling their pluripotency and differentiation potential. Here, we outline the essential role these factors play in governing the fate of stem cells and explore recent research highlighting the manipulation of epigenetic modifications to control stem cell states and differentiation.

Genetic Influence on Pluripotency and Differentiation

Genetic factors are the fundamental building blocks of an organism's DNA. They hold the blueprint for all cellular processes, including the fate of stem cells. The expression of specific genes dictates whether a stem cell remains in a pluripotent state or embarks on the path of differentiation.

For instance, transcription factors like OCT4, SOX2, and NANOG are key players in maintaining pluripotency in embryonic stem cells (ESCs). They regulate the expression of genes that keep cells in their undifferentiated state. Conversely, as stem cells commit to differentiation, specific sets of genes are turned on or off in response to environmental cues, ultimately guiding the cell toward a specialized fate.

Epigenetic Marks and Their Influence

Epigenetic modifications add another layer of complexity to stem cell regulation. These modifications, which include DNA methylation and histone modifications, don't alter the DNA sequence itself but affect how genes are accessed and expressed.

In recent years, research has revealed the pivotal role of epigenetic marks in stem cell behavior. Methylation of specific gene promoters can silence genes associated with differentiation, effectively locking stem cells in a pluripotent state. On the other hand, the removal of repressive epigenetic marks can permit the activation of lineage-specific genes, driving differentiation.

Manipulating Epigenetic Modifications

The ability to manipulate epigenetic modifications holds immense promise for stem cell research and regenerative medicine. Researchers are exploring ways to precisely control these marks to either maintain stem cell states or induce differentiation as needed.

One approach is using small molecules and genetic engineering techniques. Small molecules can target and modify specific epigenetic marks, providing a means to guide stem cell behavior. Similarly, genetic engineering tools like CRISPR-Cas9 allow for precise epigenetic editing, offering a degree of control over gene expression that was once inconceivable.

The genetic and epigenetic regulation of stem cells is a dynamic interplay that determines their pluripotency and differentiation potential. Understanding these factors is pivotal in advancing our ability to harness the therapeutic potential of stem cells. Recent research into the manipulation of epigenetic modifications offers exciting possibilities for controlling and directing the fate of these remarkable cells, opening new avenues in regenerative medicine and beyond.

Stem cell therapy is like giving the body a cellular "maintenance" crew. Because they can become almost any cell, they can theoretically go where damage and disease occurs and become the type of cell the damage and disease needs.

How does this fascinating process work?

- **Isolation and Harvesting:** Stem cells are isolated and harvested from the chosen source through minimally invasive procedures, such as bone marrow aspiration or liposuction for adipose-derived stem cells.

- **Processing and Expansion:** Once harvested, they are grown in a laboratory to increase the available quantity. This step ensures an adequate supply of stem cells for therapeutic application.

The next step is the administration of these cells into the patient's body, which can be done through injections or infusions. Once inside the body, these cells travel to the site of injury or disease and begin the repair process. The goal is for these cells to integrate with the body's natural systems and begin the healing process, whether that's by replacing diseased cells, reducing inflammation, or stimulating repair in tissues that do not regenerate easily on their own.

Success stories in stem cell therapy often read like excerpts from science fiction. For instance, in multiple sclerosis (MS) patients, stem cell transplants have been notably successful, with research revealing the therapy can reset the immune system, reducing inflammation, and preventing further myelin damage—potentially halting the progression of the disease.

Patient stories also shed light on the transformative potential of stem cell therapy. Take the example from UCLA Health's transplant program, where individuals with various blood disorders have undergone stem cell transplants. These patients, facing life-threatening illnesses like leukemia, have seen remissions and renewed hope thanks to the advanced care involving stem cells. Their stories aren't just uplifting—they're testaments to the strides being made in understanding and applying stem cell treatments.

By weaving these narratives into our exploration of stem cell therapy, we not only showcase the potential but also connect the science with the personal. These stories stand as powerful markers of progress, highlighting not only where we are but pointing to the future directions stem cell therapy might take us.

History of Stem Cell Research

The odyssey of stem cell research is a compelling tale of curiosity, dedication, and breakthroughs that have ushered in a new era in medical science. This journey traces back over a century, with roots in the late 1800s when scientists first hypothesized the existence of cells that could generate other cell types. Yet, it wasn't until the mid-20th century that these theories began to crystallize into tangible discoveries.

The first significant milestone occurred in the 1950s with the pioneering work of Canadian scientists James Till and Ernest McCulloch. They provided the first clear evidence of self-renewing cells in mice, laying the foundation for understanding stem cell principles. This breakthrough led to the identification of blood-forming stem cells in the bone marrow, revealing the potential for these cells in treating diseases such as leukemia through bone marrow transplants.

In 1981, two separate groups of researchers made history by deriving the first human embryonic stem cells. This landmark discovery unlocked a new frontier, as these cells had the capacity to become any cell type in the body, creating a dilemma for regenerative medicine.

From the 1990s to the present, stem cell research evolved rapidly. Dr. James Thomson's team at the University of Wisconsin-Madison successfully grew cells from a human embryo in the lab. This was both celebrated for its medical potential and fraught with ethical considerations, steering public discourse on the direction of stem cell research.

Amid ethical debates, scientific progress persisted. In 2006, Shinya Yamanaka developed pluripotent stem cells (iPSCs) and resolved the embryo controversy. Adult cells were changed and became able to become almost any cell. Yamanaka not only bypassed ethical issues but also opened new avenues for personalized medicine without the need for donor cells.

Technical Advances in Stem Cell Isolation and Cultivation

Over the course of the history of stem cell research, remarkable strides have been made in the field of stem cell isolation and cultivation. Regenerative medicine was developed using the new technologies.

One of the pivotal breakthroughs in stem cell research was the development of methods for isolating stem cells from various tissues and sources. Hematopoietic stem cells were isolated from bone marrow, enabling bone marrow transplants for the treatment of blood cancers. As technology progressed, scientists devised increasingly sophisticated techniques to isolate different types of stem cells from diverse tissues, such as embryonic stem cells from embryos and induced pluripotent stem cells (iPSCs) reprogrammed from adult cells. Each step forward allowed for more treatments to be considered.

Stem cell niches (discussed previously) provide the correct environment for stem cells to dwell. The niche gives signals and cues to regulate the stem cell behavior, including their self-renewal and differentiation. Understanding the intricate interplay within these niches has been pivotal in guiding researchers in their efforts to maintain stem cells in the laboratory.

However, recreating the complexity of the stem cell niche in vitro has proven to be a formidable challenge. Researchers have striven to replicate the cues from the natural niche, including biochemical signals, physical properties, and interactions with neighboring cells. While progress has been made in mimicking some aspects of these niches, fully recreating their complexity remains an ongoing pursuit. Regenerative medicine is dependent on advancing lab-grown environments to increase stem cell study.

Stem Cell Markers and Identification

Identifying stem cells from other cell types is a challenge. To overcome this hurdle, scientists rely on specific markers and molecular signatures that uniquely characterize stem cells. These markers serve as critical tools for their identification and isolation. Two primary techniques employed for this purpose are fluorescence-activated cell sorting (FACS) and magnetic-activated cell sorting (MACS).

FACS and MACS

FACS and MACS are cutting-edge methods that facilitate the isolation of stem cells based on their distinctive surface markers. FACS involves labeling cells with fluorescent antibodies targeting specific markers and then passing them through a flow cytometer. This high-tech device sorts cells based on their fluorescence, allowing researchers to collect the desired stem cell population. On the other hand, MACS employs magnetic beads coated with antibodies to bind to the target markers on cell surfaces. Magnetism is then used to separate the marked cells from the rest. Both FACS and MACS provide precise and efficient ways to isolate stem cells from complex mixtures of cells.

Marker Distinctions

Stem cell markers vary across stem cell types that we have discussed.

- **Embryonic Stem Cells (ESCs):** ESCs are known for markers like SSEA-3 (Stage-Specific Embryonic Antigen 3) and SSEA-4. These markers are associated with the pluripotent state and are prominent in the early stages of development. Additionally, the transcription factor OCT4 is a key marker involved in maintaining ESC pluripotency.

- **Adult Stem Cells:** Whether somatic or tissue-specific, stem cells exhibit different markers. For instance, hematopoietic stem cells (HSCs), which give rise to blood cells, are marked by CD34 and CD133. Mesenchymal stem cells (MSCs) commonly express markers like CD29, CD73, and CD105. These markers are specific to the tissues in which these stem cells are found and play a role in their functions.

- **Induced Pluripotent Stem Cells (iPSCs):** Discussed earlier, these are rewired adult cells. They share markers because they have been reprogrammed. OCT4, SOX2, and NANOG, among others, are used to identify iPSCs. These markers reflect the successful reprogramming of adult cells into a state resembling ESCs.

Stem cell markers are indispensable tools in the field of stem cell research, enabling scientists to precisely identify and isolate these unique cells. The markers vary depending on the type of stem cell, whether embryonic, adult, or induced pluripotent. FACS and MACS, advanced isolation techniques, play pivotal roles in harnessing the potential of stem cells for research and therapeutic applications. Understanding these markers and techniques is fundamental to advancing our knowledge and capabilities in stem cell biology.

In crafting this concise history, it is not just the cold facts of chronological events that matter, but the narrative of human endeavor. The journey of stem cell research is about the collective human effort to understand the building blocks of life with the goal of alleviating suffering and extending the quality of life. This history is still being written, as contemporary researchers stand on the shoulders of giants, striving to convert the full promise of stem cell research into treatments and therapies that could revolutionize medicine.

As we close this foundational chapter on stem cells, here are the key takeaways of what we've explored:

- Stem cells are the master cells of the body, capable of dividing and renewing themselves for long periods and differentiating into various cell types.

- Key discoveries, such as the identification of self-renewing cells in the 1950s and the derivation of human embryonic stem cells in the 1980s, have been pivotal to the advancement of stem cell research.

- Because of the controversy embryonic stem cells create, researchers searched for an alternative. The result is called pluripotent stem cells (iPSCs). These are cells created to be adaptive and offer a less controversial and more versatile source of stem cells.

- The history of stem cell research is not just a scientific chronicle but a story of ethical, legal, and social evolutions that continue to shape the field.

As we move on from the complex science and history of stem cells, we look to the horizon of what's possible. The next chapter promises to delve into the numerous conditions that stem cell therapy treats. From chronic illnesses that have long evaded cure, to acute injuries needing repair, the scope of stem cell therapy's reach is vast and holds profound implications for human health. Imagine a world where degenerative diseases no longer mean a lifetime of pain, where the damage from a heart attack is not irreversible, or where spinal cord injuries no longer result in lifelong paralysis. This is not mere fantasy; these are the horizons we're approaching through stem cell therapy. With anticipation building, we have begun exploring these applications in depth. The next chapter will not only expand your knowledge but will likely ignite your imagination, as you learn about the specific ways in which stem cell therapy is poised to redefine healing and offer new hope to millions around the globe. Stay tuned, for the journey into the potential of stem cells to heal and renew is just beginning.

Chapter 2:
Stem Cell Therapy Indications

Introduction

Stem cell therapy has created hope because of its flexibility of use. Because it has so many possibilities, it has become famous worldwide. We'll examine a variety of health conditions, including orthopedic injuries, autoimmune diseases, cardiac problems, vascular issues, and neurological disorders. We will examine case studies and research that showcase the possibilities of stem cell treatments.

Success Stories

Consider the story of Sarah, a multiple sclerosis patient who, after years of struggling with mobility issues, found renewed hope through stem cell therapy. Witness Mark, whose chronic knee pain faded into the past after a stem cell-based treatment that regenerated his joint tissues. Explore the journey of Lily, whose autoimmune disorder was managed effectively by harnessing the immune-modulating potential of stem cells.

These are just a few glimpses into the stories of lives changed by stem cell therapy. They stand as testament to the versatility and promise of this groundbreaking field of medicine. Stem cell therapy isn't confined to a single ailment; rather, it has the potential to touch the lives of countless patients facing a wide range of health challenges.

Generalized Conditions Treated with Stem Cell Therapy

These cells can become various cell types. Thus, they can replace many different damaged or diseased cells. Let's take a closer look at the categories of conditions treated with stem cell therapy:

- Neurological Disorders such as Parkinson's disease, Alzheimer's disease, amyotrophic lateral sclerosis (ALS), and spinal cord injuries have been impossible to cure. Symptom relief is not even very effective. Studies utilizing stem cell therapy are showing some positive results although we are far from cures currently.

- Stem cell therapy shows potential in treating orthopedic injuries and age-related conditions like osteoarthritis, cartilage problems, and tendon damage. Joint tissues, including cartilage and ligaments, can be healed leading to greater mobility and pain relief.

- Autoimmune diseases like rheumatoid arthritis, multiple sclerosis, and lupus involve the immune system attacking the body's own tissues. Disease progression and symptom relief show improvement with stem cell therapies in early studies.

- Ischemic heart disease, congestive heart failure, and peripheral artery disease could potentially improve by enhancing heart function with stem cell treatments.

Stem cell therapy's scope extends well beyond these categories, with ongoing research exploring its potential for treating a wide array of other conditions, including diabetes, pulmonary diseases, liver disorders, and specific types of cancer. As research progresses, the range of potential applications for stem cells continues to expand.

Treating Neurological Disorders with Stem Cell Therapy

Parkinson's Disease

Parkinson's disease is characterized by the degeneration of dopamine-producing brain cells leading to motor deficits. Dopamine-producing nerve cells are created from stem cells and are then placed into affected brain cells.

A notable success story in this realm is the groundbreaking milestone achieved by Lund University, where the first patient received a stem cell-based transplant for Parkinson's disease (Lund University, 2023). This pioneering approach aims to replace the lost neurons and restore dopamine production. Additional research is needed, but this demonstrates the potential for improvement in Parkinson's patients.

Alzheimer's Disease

Alzheimer's disease, a devastating neurodegenerative disorder, has proven to be a formidable challenge. Recent studies have explored the transplantation of neural stem cells or their derivatives to replace damaged brain cells and potentially slow down the disease's progression.

Though the field is still in its infancy, researchers are optimistic about the potential of stem cell therapy in addressing

Alzheimer's disease. Ongoing investigations are shedding light on the intricate mechanisms involved, offering hope for future treatments.

Spinal Cord Injuries

Spinal cord damage can possibly be healed with stem cell treatments. Recent studies have examined the transplantation of neural stem cells, mesenchymal stem cells, or induced pluripotent stem cell-derived neural cells into injured spinal cords.

While not a guaranteed cure, these studies have shown promise in terms of motor function improvement and sensory recovery. One example is recent research which highlights the potential of stem cell-based approaches in spinal cord injury treatment (Zeng, 2023).

Recent breakthroughs and ongoing research provide a glimpse into a future where these conditions may become more manageable, offering hope to countless individuals and their families. While challenges remain, the progress in the field of stem cell therapy continues to inspire optimism and a renewed sense of possibility for those affected by neurological disorders.

Stem Cell Therapy in Orthopedics

Orthopedic conditions, which encompass joint pain, osteoarthritis, and cartilage injuries, have long been a source of discomfort and reduced mobility for many individuals. Stem cell therapy holds promise in addressing these orthopedic challenges. In this section, we will explore the use of stem cell therapy in orthopedics, backed by clinical trials and outcomes that shed light on its potential.

Treating Joint Pain

Joint pain, often caused by wear and tear, injury, or inflammation, can significantly impact an individual's quality of life. Researchers have been studying a type of stem cell called mesenchymal stem cells (MSCs) for this purpose. These cells can change into different cell types, including cartilage cells (chondrocytes) and bone-forming cells (osteoblasts). This characteristic makes MSCs particularly well-suited for addressing joint pain and related orthopedic conditions. By injecting MSCs into the affected joint, they can contribute to tissue repair and regeneration, potentially alleviating pain and improving joint function. Studies show that stem cells are helpful for relieving joint pain.

Osteoarthritis Management

Osteoarthritis, a common orthopedic condition characterized by the gradual degeneration of joint cartilage, presents a significant challenge in the medical field. Stem cell therapy holds promise as a potential intervention. Recent studies have explored the use of stem cells, particularly MSCs, to stimulate cartilage repair and slow down the progression of osteoarthritis.

The goal is to enhance cartilage regeneration and reduce inflammation by injecting stem cells into the joint. While research in this area is ongoing, the preliminary results have shown promise in improving joint function and reducing pain.

Cartilage Injuries and Repair

Cartilage injuries, whether due to sports-related trauma or degenerative conditions, can have a lasting impact on an individual's mobility and comfort. By delivering stem cells directly to the site of cartilage damage, researchers aim to stimulate the repair and growth of healthy cartilage tissue.

Clinical trials for cartilage repair typically involve the isolation and expansion of MSCs from the patient's own tissues, followed by their transplantation into the injured area. These trials have demonstrated encouraging outcomes, with some patients experiencing significant improvements in pain relief and joint function.

Clinical trials have provided valuable evidence of its potential effectiveness in improving joint function, reducing pain, and promoting tissue regeneration. While further research is needed to refine techniques and optimize outcomes, the field of stem cell therapy in orthopedics continues to offer hope for individuals seeking relief from orthopedic challenges.

Autoimmune Diseases

Autoimmune conditions arise from the immune system targeting the body's tissues. They are difficult to treat. Tissue repair using stem cells has ignited fresh hope for multiple sclerosis, rheumatoid arthritis, and lupus.

Potential for Treating Autoimmune Diseases

The mesenchymal stem cells possess the ability to modulate and regulate the immune response, offering a potential solution to rein in the overactive immune system responsible for autoimmune attacks.

Immune-Modulating Properties of Stem Cells

MSCs coming from bone marrow or adipose tissue have been a focus of research in the context of autoimmune diseases. These cells have the remarkable capacity to suppress inflammatory immune responses while promoting regulatory immune cells that maintain tolerance and prevent excessive immune reactions.

When introduced into the body, MSCs can act as immune system moderators. They can reduce the harmful effects of autoimmune attacks by releasing anti-inflammatory molecules, preventing further tissue damage, and promoting tissue repair. This unique property makes them a potential therapeutic tool for managing autoimmune conditions.

Real-World Applications and Success Stories

Sarah's journey with multiple sclerosis (MS) had been a long and arduous one. For years, she grappled with the debilitating effects of this autoimmune disorder, which had slowly but steadily eroded her quality of life. MS had taken its toll on her body, leaving her with symptoms that made everyday activities challenging and painful. Walking had become a struggle, and fatigue was a constant companion. The unpredictability of MS exacerbations was emotionally taxing, making it difficult for Sarah to plan her life with any sense of certainty.

With the challenges, Sarah held onto a glimmer of hope. She learned about stem cell therapy improving MS and other autoimmune disorders. Sarah decided to explore this option, hoping it could bring some relief to her life.

After consulting with her healthcare team, Sarah embarked on a journey towards stem cell therapy. The procedure involved the infusion of mesenchymal stem cells, which are known for their regenerative and immunomodulatory properties. These cells had the potential to reset her immune system, calming the overactive responses that were responsible for the damage caused by MS.

The process was not without its challenges and uncertainties. Sarah and her medical team carefully discussed the potential risks and benefits of the therapy, ensuring she had a clear understanding of what to expect. While stem cell therapy held great promise, it was not a guaranteed cure, and results could vary from person to person.

Over time, Sarah noticed changes. Her symptoms, which had once been relentless, started to stabilize. Fatigue no longer dominated her days, and she found herself regaining some of her lost mobility. Walking became less of a struggle, and her overall quality of life improved significantly. The unpredictability of MS relapses became less daunting, and Sarah could finally make plans with greater confidence.

Sarah's story serves as a powerful example of the potential of stem cell therapy in managing autoimmune disorders. While it may not be a standardized solution, it offers hope and a chance at a better quality of life for individuals like her. Stem cells, with their remarkable ability to modulate the immune system and promote healing, bring hope in the battle against autoimmune diseases. Sarah's journey is a testament to the ongoing advancements in medical science and the resilience of those who refuse to surrender to the challenges of chronic illness.

Clinical trials and studies have also contributed to our understanding of stem cell therapy's potential in autoimmune diseases. While research is ongoing, outcomes have shown positive trends, with many patients experiencing reduced disease activity and improved symptoms.

Real-world cases and ongoing research underscore the promise of this innovative avenue in providing relief and hope to individuals grappling with autoimmune disorders. While challenges remain, the potential of stem cell therapy continues to inspire optimism and exploration in the field of autoimmune disease management.

Cardiac and Vascular Conditions

Cardiac and vascular conditions, such as myocardial infarction (heart attack) and peripheral artery disease, represent significant challenges in the field of medicine. Repairing heart and blood vessels can be accomplished with stem cell treatments. In this section, we will examine the applications of stem cell therapy in cardiac and vascular conditions, explaining the current standard of care and how stem cell therapy could enhance treatment outcomes.

Myocardial Infarction

In myocardial infarction (heart attack) heart tissue death occurs from a blocked artery of the heart's blood supply. There is usually impaired cardiac function. The current standard of care for myocardial infarction typically involves interventions like angioplasty and stent placement to restore blood flow and the use of medications to manage symptoms.

The idea is to introduce stem cells, often derived from the patient's own tissues, into the damaged heart tissue. The cells become cardiomyocytes (heart muscle cells), and release factors that stimulate tissue healing.

Clinical studies and research have shown promising results, with some patients experiencing improved cardiac function and reduced scar tissue after stem cell therapy. While further research is needed to refine techniques and optimize outcomes, stem cell therapy holds the potential to enhance the recovery of heart attack survivors.

Peripheral Artery Disease (PAD)

Atherosclerosis causes blood vessels to narrow, commonly in legs. This condition can lead to reduced blood flow, claudication (pain while walking), and in severe cases, tissue damage and limb amputation. Current standard treatments for PAD include lifestyle changes, medications, and, in advanced cases, surgical interventions such as angioplasty or bypass surgery.

Stem cell therapy addresses PAD by stimulating vascular regeneration. Mesenchymal stem cells (MSCs) and other stem cell types have demonstrated the ability to enhance blood vessel formation and improve blood flow in preclinical and clinical studies. The cells are delivered directly to the affected areas, promoting angiogenesis (the formation of new blood vessels) and alleviating the symptoms of PAD.

While research in this field is ongoing, the potential of stem cell therapy to improve blood circulation and reduce the need for invasive surgical procedures holds promise for individuals with peripheral artery disease.

The treatment of cardiac and vascular conditions can be revolutionized. By harnessing the regenerative power of stem cells, researchers hope to promote cardiac repair and vascular regeneration, offering hope for improved outcomes and a better quality of life for patients grappling with these conditions. The potential benefits are impressive.

Stem Cell Therapy in Other Conditions

Stem cell therapy is being studied for many other diseases and disorders. We will discuss some of them here.

Diabetes

Diabetes is a common disease worldwide. Islet cells in the pancreas are not able to secrete insulin normally, or at all in the case of type 1 diabetes. Restoring pancreatic cells is being studied. The goal is to restore normal insulin production and glucose regulation. While research is ongoing, this approach holds potential for individuals living with diabetes.

Pulmonary Diseases

Here's a brief overview of the potential use of stem cell therapy for certain severe pulmonary diseases:

- **Chronic obstructive pulmonary disease (COPD):** Stem cell therapy, particularly mesenchymal stem cell

(MSC) therapy, has shown promise in preclinical studies and early clinical trials for COPD. It may have anti-inflammatory and regenerative effects on damaged lung tissue.

- **Asthma:** Stem cell-based approaches, such as using mesenchymal stem cells, are being investigated for severe, difficult-to-treat asthma cases. These cells reduce inflammation and modulate the immune response.

- **Interstitial Lung Disease (ILD):** Some studies are exploring stem cell therapy, including the use of mesenchymal stem cells, for ILD. Research is ongoing to determine its safety and efficacy.

- **Pulmonary Hypertension:** Stem cell therapy is being studied for its potential to improve pulmonary hypertension by promoting blood vessel repair and reducing pulmonary artery pressure.

- **Cystic Fibrosis:** While gene therapy is a primary focus for cystic fibrosis, stem cell research may offer alternative approaches in the future for repairing damaged lung tissue.

- **Idiopathic Pulmonary Fibrosis (IPF):** Stem cell therapies, including the use of MSCs and lung tissue engineering, are being explored as potential treatments for IPF.

- **Bronchiectasis:** Stem cell-based approaches may have potential in repairing damaged airways in bronchiectasis patients.

It's important to emphasize that stem cell therapy is not a standardized or approved treatment for most severe pulmonary diseases currently.

Liver Disorders

Liver disorders such as cirrhosis and liver failure can have life-threatening consequences. Damaged liver cells are treated with stem cells that become like liver cells. While research is still in its infancy, this approach holds potential for addressing liver diseases and reducing the need for liver transplantation.

Cancer Treatment

Stem cell therapy is also finding applications in cancer treatment, particularly in the context of hematopoietic stem cell transplantation. These treatments aim to replace or repair damaged bone marrow cells in patients undergoing aggressive cancer treatments like chemotherapy or radiation. By restoring healthy blood cell production, stem cell therapy plays a crucial role in managing and relieving the side effects of cancer treatments.

While these are just a few examples, the potential of stem cell therapy in addressing a wide range of health conditions continues to expand. Innovative treatments become closer to common medical practice with continuing research and treatment trials.

Future Directions in Stem Cell Therapy

As we look forward, we can anticipate exciting advancements and new horizons. The following are areas of interest:

- **Personalized Medicine:** An individual's genetic and medical profiles are used to develop specific therapies. This approach ensures that patients receive the most effective and customized therapies, maximizing treatment success.

- **Tissue Engineering:** Stem cell therapy will play a pivotal role in tissue engineering, where artificial organs and tissues are created using a patient's own stem cells. This holds great promise for patients in need of organ transplants and those with tissue damage or degenerative conditions.

- **Combining Therapies:** Researchers are studying the effects of blending current therapies with stem cells. Treatments such as gene therapy or immunotherapy could be enhanced to target a broader range of conditions.

- **Regulations:** Creating strong regulatory structures and guidelines is vital to guarantee the safe and morally sound progression of stem cell treatments. These frameworks will guide clinical trials, treatment protocols, and patient safety.

Revealing the Potential of Stem Cell Therapy

As our understanding of stem cell research increases, the horizons of possibilities seem boundless. In this section, we will speculate on the future directions of stem cell research, including the potential development of organ regeneration, the creation of bioartificial organs, and the intriguing theoretical concept of "de-aging" stem cells and its implications for life extension research.

Organ Regeneration

One of the most tantalizing prospects on the horizon of stem cell research is the development of organ regeneration. Imagine a future where damaged or failing organs can be repaired or replaced with newly grown, fully functional ones. This vision is not as far-fetched as it may seem.

Researchers are actively working on methods to coax stem cells into forming specific organs, paving the way for organ regeneration. Already, there have been successful experiments in growing miniature organs, known as organoids, in the lab. These organoids mimic the structure and function of real organs, providing valuable tools for studying diseases and potential treatments.

In the future, it is plausible that scientists will refine these techniques to create full-sized, functional organs for transplantation. This would revolutionize organ transplantation, eliminating the need for donors and the risk of rejection, ultimately saving countless lives.

Bioartificial Organs

Going hand in hand with organ regeneration is the concept of bioartificial organs. In addition to growing new organs from stem cells, researchers are exploring the development of artificial organs that can mimic the form and function of natural ones.

These bioartificial organs may consist of a scaffold made from biocompatible materials, seeded with patient-specific stem cells. Over time, the stem cells would differentiate and populate the scaffold, creating an organ that is personalized to the patient's genetic makeup, reducing the risk of rejection. Bioartificial organs hold immense potential not only for transplantation but also for serving as temporary solutions while patients await natural organ regeneration.

"De-Aging" Stem Cells and Life Extension

In the realm of theoretical applications, an intriguing concept emerges—the "de-aging" of stem cells. While currently theoretical and largely speculative, this concept suggests that stem cells could be manipulated to reset or rejuvenate the biological clock, effectively reversing the aging process in certain tissues or organs.

The implications of such a breakthrough would be profound, not only in terms of aesthetic benefits but also for extending healthy human lifespan. Imagine a future where stem cells could be used to repair age-related damage to the heart, brain, or other vital organs, effectively delaying the onset of age-related diseases and extending the period of vitality and productivity.

This concept serves as a tantalizing glimpse into the potential of stem cells to redefine the boundaries of aging and longevity research.

Challenges and Ethical Considerations

Of course, with these future directions and theoretical advances come significant challenges and ethical considerations. The ethical implications of creating bioartificial organs or manipulating stem cells for life extension are complex and require careful consideration. Issues such as consent, equitable access, and the potential for misuse must be addressed as these technologies advance.

Furthermore, the scientific hurdles are not insignificant. Stem cell research requires rigorous safety testing and validation before new therapies can be implemented. The risk of unintended consequences or unexpected side effects must be carefully studied and removed.

The future of stem cell research is a tantalizing landscape of possibilities. From organ regeneration to bioartificial organs and the theoretical concept of "de-aging" stem cells, the potential benefits are immense. However, along with these opportunities come ethical and scientific challenges that must be addressed carefully. As we continue to explore these uncharted territories, the remarkable versatility and regenerative potential of stem cells hold the promise of transforming healthcare and extending the boundaries of human health and longevity. The journey is just beginning, and the future of stem cell research is a frontier awaiting exploration.

Chapter 3:
Types of Stem Cell Therapy

The capacity to combine the knowledge of genes with the potential of stem cells opens up exciting possibilities for personalized medicine. —James A. Thomson

In the previous chapters, we ventured into the world of stem cell therapy, uncovering its remarkable potential to transform healthcare. Now we will explore the various types of stem cell therapies currently available, including autologous, allogeneic, and induced pluripotent stem cells (iPSCs). We will provide an overview of each of these therapies, their applications, and potential challenges, shedding light on the multifaceted nature of this groundbreaking field.

Autologous Stem Cell Therapy

Autologous stem cell therapy represents a pioneering approach in regenerative medicine, one that taps into the body's innate capacity for healing and rejuvenation. In this section, we will provide an in-depth exploration of what autologous stem cell therapy entails, shedding light on the procedures involved, potential benefits, drawbacks, and ethical considerations.

Understanding Autologous Stem Cell Therapy

These stem cells come directly from the patient, typically from one of the following sources:

- **Bone Marrow:** This is one of the most common sources for autologous stem cell therapy. A small quantity of bone marrow is aspirated from the patient's hip bone, usually under local anesthesia.

- **Fatty Tissue:** Fat, also called adipose tissue, (unfortunately) found in abundance, is a source for mesenchymal stem cells (MSCs). A minor liposuction procedure is used to collect the fat tissue.

- **Peripheral Blood:** A patient's blood is processed through a machine, collecting the stem cells then returning the blood to the body.

The Procedure

- **Harvesting:** The first step in autologous stem cell therapy is the collection of the patient's stem cells from the chosen source. The choice of source depends on the condition being treated.

- **Processing:** The stem cells are isolated and concentrated. This step ensures that the therapy is as effective as possible.

- **Reintroduction:** After processing, the concentrated stem cells are reintroduced into the patient's body, often through targeted injections or infusions. The goal is to deliver these cells to the site of injury or disease, where they can exert their regenerative effects.

Potential Benefits

- **Compatibility:** Since the cells used belong to the patient, there is minimal risk of immune rejection or allergic reactions.

- **Regeneration:** Cells differentiate into many cell types so can be used on multiple tissues.

- **Safety:** Has a low risk of adverse effects and is considered safer.

Autologous stem cell therapy challenges and ethical considerations:

- **Cell Viability:** The quality and quantity of a patient's own stem cells may vary, particularly with age. This variability can impact treatment outcomes.

- **Patient Safety:** The harvesting process, while generally safe, can carry risks associated with anesthesia or minor surgical procedures.

- **Ethical Concerns:** Although autologous therapy bypasses many ethical concerns associated with other stem cell sources, questions related to informed consent and the responsible use of these therapies remain relevant.

- **Real-World Impact:** Autologous stem cell therapy has made significant strides in a number of medical fields. It can be used to treat everything from joint pain and arthritis, to damaged heart tissue. Additionally, autologous stem cell therapy has found applications in dermatology, neurology, and more.

Treatments

Treatments are developed using the patient's cells. Stem cells are typically harvested from blood, fatty tissue or bone marrow. The treatments are varied and listed below:

- **Orthopedic Injuries:** Autologous stem cells are often injected directly into the affected area, promoting tissue repair, and reducing pain.

- **Cardiac Conditions:** Damaged heart muscle (such as after a heart attack) improves with stem cell treatment, as does heart function.

- **Neurological Disorders:** Some neurological conditions, such as spinal cord injuries and multiple sclerosis, have been the focus of autologous stem cell research. The hope is that these cells can promote nerve regeneration and alleviate symptoms.

- **Dermatological Applications:** Autologous stem cells have also been explored in the field of dermatology for wound healing and skin rejuvenation.

While autologous stem cell therapy is promising, it is not without challenges. One significant limitation is that the quantity and quality of a patient's own stem cells may vary, particularly as individuals age. Additionally, the harvesting process can be invasive and may not be suitable for all patients. This treatment is limited based on availability of cell sources.

Allogeneic Stem Cell Therapy

Allogeneic stem cell therapy represents a remarkable leap in regenerative medicine, offering the potential for life-saving treatments by utilizing stem cells from a carefully matched donor.

The Procedure

Allogeneic stem cells come from a donor. This donor could be a family member, an unrelated individual, or even cord blood from a public bank. The critical aspect here is meticulous matching to reduce the risk of complications.

The Matching Process

Matching donors and recipients in allogeneic stem cell therapy is a complex but crucial process. Immunological considerations take center stage in this endeavor. A donor is found who has human leukocyte antigen (HLA) markers closely matching those of the recipient. HLA markers are essential for immune system function, and a close match minimizes the risk of graft-versus-host disease (GVHD)—a potentially severe complication where the donor's immune cells attack the recipient's tissues.

Allogeneic stem cell therapy offers several potential advantages:

- **Disease Eradication:** It is particularly effective in treating hematologic malignancies like leukemia and lymphoma, where the goal is to eliminate cancerous cells through high-dose chemotherapy and radiation followed by the infusion of healthy donor stem cells.

- **Donor Graft Effect:** The donor's immune cells can recognize and attack cancer cells in the recipient, enhancing the anti-cancer effect known as the graft-versus-leukemia (GVL) or graft-versus-tumor (GVT) effect.

- **Broader Applicability:** Allogeneic therapy is suitable for patients who may not have sufficient or healthy autologous stem cells, such as those with genetic conditions or extensive prior treatments.

While allogeneic stem cell therapy holds tremendous promise, it is not without limitations:

- **GVHD Risk:** The risk of GVHD, where the donor immune cells attack the recipient's tissues, can be significant. Immunosuppressive medications are used to mitigate this risk but may have side effects.

- **Matching Challenges:** Finding a suitable donor with compatible HLA markers can be challenging, particularly for patients from diverse racial or ethnic backgrounds.

- **Immunosuppression:** Patients receiving allogeneic therapy require ongoing immunosuppressive medications to prevent rejection of the donor cells. There is an increased risk of infection and other complications.

Applications

Hematopoietic Stem Cell Transplantation (HSCT)

Allogeneic HSCT is a well-established treatment for various blood-related disorders, including leukemia, lymphoma, and sickle cell anemia. It involves replacing a patient's diseased blood-forming stem cells with healthy ones from a matching donor.

Immunotherapy

Allogeneic immune cell therapies, such as chimeric antigen receptor (CAR) T-cell therapy, have gained prominence in cancer treatment. In this approach, engineered immune cells from a donor are used to target and destroy cancer cells in the recipient's body.

Mesenchymal Stem Cell Therapies

Allogeneic mesenchymal stem cells (MSCs) are being investigated for their potential to treat conditions like graft-versus-host disease (GVHD), an immune system response that can occur after allogeneic HSCT. Allogeneic MSCs may also be used for orthopedic and inflammatory conditions.

Allogeneic Stem Cell Therapy

Allogeneic stem cell therapy has revolutionized the treatment of various hematologic and immunologic conditions. In hematologic oncology, it is a frontline treatment for leukemia, lymphoma, and other blood cancers. Additionally, allogeneic stem cell therapy has expanded its reach into treating non-malignant conditions like aplastic anemia and certain immune disorders.

While allogeneic stem cell therapy offers broader availability of cell sources and potentially more robust treatments, it comes with challenges related to immune compatibility and the risk of graft-versus-host reactions. Careful donor selection and matching are crucial to minimize these risks.

Induced Pluripotent Stem Cells (iPSCs)

Induced pluripotent stem cells (iPSCs) stand as a testament to the remarkable progress in stem cell research, offering a unique avenue for harnessing the body's regenerative potential. These cells are produced by retraining. Adult skin or blood cells are turned into a flexible state, similar to embryonic stem cells.

Creating iPSCs: A Breakthrough in Cellular Reprogramming

The creation of iPSCs represents a groundbreaking achievement in the field of stem cell biology. iPSCs are not collected but rather created via cellular reprogramming. This innovative procedure involves the conversion of fully developed, specialized cells like skin cells or blood cells back into a pluripotent state. As discussed previously, these cells can form into almost any cell type of the body.

The discovery of iPSCs was first pioneered by Shinya Yamanaka and John B. Gurdon in 2006, and they were awarded the Nobel Prize in Physiology or Medicine in 2012. Their investigation paved the way for the creation of patient-tailored stem cells, alleviating the ethical dilemmas often linked to embryonic stem cells.

Applications of iPSCs: Unleashing Regenerative Potential

- **Disease Modeling:** Cellular models of various diseases are recreated then studied in the lab. Those most studied are the mechanisms of disease, drug development, and personalized therapies targeting specific receptor sites.

- **Cell Replacement Therapy:** iPSCs can be differentiated into specific cell types needed for transplantation, offering a potential source of replacement cells for conditions like Parkinson's disease, diabetes, and spinal cord injuries.

- **Drug Testing:** iPSC-derived cells enable more accurate and personalized drug testing, potentially reducing adverse drug reactions and improving drug efficacy.

- **Understanding Development:** iPSCs offer insights into early human development and embryogenesis, shedding light on the formation of tissues and organs.

While iPSCs hold immense promise, several challenges must be addressed.

- **Tumor Formation:** iPSCs have the potential to form tumors if they are not fully reprogrammed or if they differentiate into unintended cell types. Ensuring their safety for therapeutic use remains a critical concern.

- **Reprogramming Efficiency:** The process of reprogramming cells into iPSCs is still relatively inefficient and time-consuming, requiring optimization for broader clinical applications.

- **Ethical Questions:** While iPSCs bypass some ethical concerns associated with embryonic stem cells, they raise their own set of ethical questions related to the use of patient-specific cells and consent.

Despite their remarkable potential, iPSCs face challenges related to safety, quality control, and the potential for tumorigenicity (the formation of tumors). Research efforts are ongoing to address these concerns and harness the full therapeutic potential of iPSCs.

All of these therapies offer unique advantages and applications across many conditions. However, each type also comes with its own set of challenges and considerations, from immune compatibility to safety and tumorigenicity concerns.

As we explore the dynamic landscape of stem cell research, iPSCs stand at the forefront of scientific innovation. They hold the potential to revolutionize medicine by offering personalized treatments, deeper insights into disease mechanisms, and enhanced drug development processes. We will examine the specific applications of iPSCs in various medical fields, witnessing firsthand how these reprogrammed cells are shaping the future of healthcare. From neurological disorders to cardiac conditions, iPSCs are paving the way for a new era in regenerative medicine, where the power to heal lies within the very cells that make us who we are.

Challenges Faced in Stem Cell Research

- **Safety and Efficacy:** Rigorous clinical trials and regulatory oversight are necessary to validate these treatments and protect patient well-being.

- **Ethical Considerations:** The use of embryonic stem cells causes ethical outrage related to the source of these cells and their use in research and therapy. Striking a balance between scientific advancement and ethical principles remains an ongoing challenge.

- **Standardization:** Achieving consistency and standardization in stem cell therapies is essential. Variability in cell sources, preparation methods, and quality control can impact treatment outcomes. Developing industry-wide standards is crucial for reliable therapies.

- **Immune Compatibility:** For allogeneic stem cell therapies, immune compatibility and the risk of graft-versus-host reactions must be carefully managed. Matching donors to recipients is critical, and research into immune tolerance is ongoing.

- **Tumorigenicity:** The potential for stem cells, especially iPSCs, to form tumors or other unwanted cell types is a significant concern. Ensuring the safety of these therapies is a complex challenge.

- **Regulatory Approval:** The road to regulatory approval for stem cell therapies can be lengthy and arduous. Demonstrating safety and efficacy through clinical trials and navigating regulatory pathways is a substantial undertaking for researchers and developers.

- **Accessibility:** Ensuring equitable access to stem cell therapies is crucial. Addressing issues of cost, availability, and disparities in healthcare access is an ongoing challenge in realizing the full potential of these treatments.

As we discuss the specifics of stem cell therapies in the chapters ahead, it is essential to keep these challenges in mind. Stem cell research is a dynamic field, continually evolving to address these hurdles and refine therapies. With each new discovery, the potential to alleviate suffering, improve lives, and push the boundaries of medicine draws closer.

The world of stem cell therapies offers a vast array of possibilities and potential benefits. However, it is equally crucial to understand that not all stem cell treatments are created equal. In the next chapter, we will equip you with the essential tools to critically evaluate claims about stem cell therapy, ensuring that you can make informed decisions. Join us on a journey to understand stem cell treatments, separating fact from fiction in regenerative medicine.

Chapter 4:
Evaluating Stem Cell Therapy

The Promise and Perils of Regenerative Medicine

Stem cell therapies hold the promise of revolutionary breakthroughs in healthcare, offering hope to countless individuals grappling with debilitating conditions. The potential to regenerate damaged tissue and organs, alleviate suffering, and enhance the quality of life is an enticing prospect. Yet, with this tantalizing promise, a sobering truth emerges—stem cell therapies have both immense potential and grave peril.

Serious Safety Concerns With Regenerative Medicine

Safety concerns surrounding stem cell therapies have cast a long and sometimes ominous shadow over this field. The allure of regenerating tissues and reversing diseases has prompted a proliferation of clinics and treatments, some of which may not meet the rigorous standards necessary for patient safety. In the past, patients have experienced devastating consequences when subjected to unproven and inadequately regulated stem cell interventions.

The U.S. Food and Drug Administration (FDA), in a stern warning, cautions about the dangers of stem cell therapies (Santhosh, 2024). Their message is clear: While there are legitimate and promising stem cell treatments, there are also charlatans and unscrupulous actors who put patients at risk with unproven and potentially dangerous interventions.

As we evaluate stem cell therapies, we must recognize the gravity of the safety concerns of this field. This chapter will provide you with the tools, knowledge, and critical insights needed to evaluate stem cell treatments.

The Path Ahead

In this chapter, we will outline the evaluation of stem cell therapies. We will assess various crucial factors:

- **Understanding the Benefits:** We will begin with the potential benefits and the remarkable results that stem cell therapy can offer to patients. From neurological disorders to cardiac conditions, we will witness firsthand the transformative potential of these treatments.

- **Safety Considerations:** Safety is paramount when considering any medical intervention. We will dissect the safety concerns associated with stem cell therapies, including the risks and complications that must be weighed alongside their potential benefits.

- **Clinical Trials:** The backbone of evidence-based medicine, clinical trials are the litmus test for the efficacy and safety of stem cell therapies. We will explore clinical trials, providing insights into their significance and what to look for when assessing their outcomes.

- **Regulations and Legalities:** Stem cell therapies operate under regulations and laws that vary by country.

We will explain the standards and guidelines that govern these treatments.

You will learn how to evaluate stem cell therapies, critically assess claims about stem cell treatments and make informed decisions about your health or the health of your loved ones.

Benefits and Potential Outcomes

To understand stem cell therapies, it is essential to first understand the benefits and potential outcomes that have captivated the imaginations of patients and medical professionals alike.

Unlike traditional treatments that merely manage symptoms, stem cell therapy addresses the root causes of various medical conditions, paving the way for genuine healing and restoration.

A Multitude of Conditions

Stem Cell Therapy: A Rising Tide brings us the insights of Dr. Neil Riordan, a renowned scientist and pioneer in the field of stem cell therapy (Riordan, 2017). Dr. Riordan first explored the pro-oxidant effects of high-dose intravenous vitamin C on cancer. This led to the development of the mesenchymal stem cell technologies that he currently uses at the Stem Cell Institute in Panama.

In an interview, Dr. Riordan discusses his early research career, where he made a remarkable discovery—high doses of vitamin C could elevate blood levels to a point where the vitamin could effectively target and kill cancer cells (Riordan, 2017). This breakthrough had significant implications for cancer treatment.

The subsequent exploration of dendritic cells as part of immune system stimulation opened doors to stem cell research.

Dr. Riordan's work with stem cells began with the aspiration to enhance dendritic cell vaccines further. To achieve this, patients were given a drug called G-CSF to stimulate the production of stem cells in their bone marrow. These stem cells were then converted into dendritic cells to create more potent therapeutic vaccines.

Dr. Riordan provides insights into the different types of stem cells found in various body sites and how to support and nurture tissue-specific stem cells. His research primarily focuses on MSCs and their ability to stimulate healing through their secretions.

What sets MSCs apart is their remarkable capacity to address a wide range of chronic diseases by modulating inflammation, regulating the immune system, and promoting tissue regeneration. Dr. Riordan's work has revealed that many chronic diseases result from a lack or dysfunction of MSCs, making these cells a promising avenue for treatment.

He stresses using adult stem cells acquired from uncontentious sources. Dr. Riordan advocates for the responsible use of stem cells to maximize their healing potential.

Finally, he highlights the conditions that can be treated with autologous bone marrow mesenchymal stem cells, including multiple sclerosis, Duchenne muscular dystrophy, spinal cord injuries, and various other orthopedic, cardiac, and neurological disorders. The beneficial effects seem to appear fairly quickly. While the specific timeline for improvement varies depending on the condition and individual response, many patients report noticeable benefits within weeks to months after treatment.

Dr. Neil Riordan's work in stem cell therapy offers hope for individuals suffering from chronic diseases. His groundbreaking research has paved the way for innovative treatments, and his dedication to responsible and ethical stem cell use sets a positive example for the field. Dr. Riordan's research shows stem cell therapy offers the ability to treat numerous diseases.

With ethical considerations at the forefront, Dr. Riordan's work serves as a testament to responsible and groundbreaking research in the field of regenerative medicine.

Whether you're a patient, a healthcare professional, or simply someone curious about the science of stem cells, we should all strive for a future where diseases are only a hurdle, not a dead end. Together, through informed decisions and scientific advancements, we can help shape the future of medicine. Our exploration of the upcoming chapters will provide further insights into the complex yet promising world of stem cell therapy.

Stories of Transformation

Consider Lila, a 45-year-old woman with osteoarthritis in her knees, who had been struggling with chronic pain and limited mobility. After undergoing stem cell therapy, she noticed a significant reduction in pain within a few weeks. Over the following months, her joint function improved, allowing her to enjoy activities she had long abandoned.

Similarly, Mark, a 55-year-old man diagnosed with multiple sclerosis, experienced recurrent relapses, and worsening symptoms. Stem cell therapy offered him a glimmer of hope. While it didn't provide an instant cure, Mark observed a decrease in relapses and improved daily functioning over the course of a year after treatment.

These stories exemplify the potential for stem cell therapy to transform lives, offering a renewed sense of hope and a path towards improved well-being. However, it's crucial to acknowledge that not all patients experience such dramatic outcomes, and results can vary widely.

Autologous Stem Cell Therapy: A Safer Option?

Autologous stem cell therapy, which utilizes a patient's own stem cells, is often perceived as safer than other types of stem cell therapy due to reduced concerns about immune rejection. However, there are other risks that need to be considered.

1. **Infection Risk:** A potential concern linked with autologous stem cell therapy pertains to the risk of infection. The process of harvesting and handling stem cells carries the potential for contamination. Patients receive treatments in a sterile environment to minimize this risk.

2. **Procedural Risks:** The harvesting of stem cells, particularly bone marrow or adipose tissue, involves a medical procedure that carries its own set of risks. Infection, bleeding, and damage to surrounding tissues are potential complications.

3. **Lack of Efficacy:** While autologous stem cell therapy is generally considered safe in terms of immune compatibility, it may not always deliver the desired therapeutic outcomes. Lack of efficacy may be related

to the disease being treated, the patient's health, and the quality of the stem cells.

4. **Short-Term Side Effects:** Short-term side effects such as pain, swelling, or discomfort at the injection or harvesting site are common but typically resolve within a few days to weeks.

Allogeneic Stem Cell Therapy: Balancing Potential Benefits and Risks

Because this therapy uses cells that are foreign to the patient, allogeneic therapy has other risks:

Immune Response and Graft-versus-Host Disease (GVHD)

Because the cells come from another person, there is a chance for an immune response in the recipient. If the donor cells are not closely matched to the recipient's human leukocyte antigen (HLA) markers, it can lead to graft-versus-host disease (GVHD). GVHD is a severe condition where the donor's immune cells attack the recipient's tissues. To mitigate this risk, meticulous matching is crucial, and immunosuppressive medications are often used post-transplant.

Infection Risk

Patients receiving allogeneic stem cell transplants are at an increased risk of infections, as their immune systems are temporarily suppressed to prevent rejection of the donor cells.

Long-Term Risks

Long-term risks associated with allogeneic stem cell therapy may include chronic GVHD, which can affect various organs and systems in the body. Additionally, patients may require ongoing immunosuppressive medications, which can have their own set of side effects and risks.

The Unknowns and the Need for Rigorous Research

There are still unknowns and uncertainties that underscore the importance of rigorous research and clinical trials. The field is evolving rapidly, and as new therapies emerge, their safety profiles must be thoroughly examined.

Unknown Long-Term Effects

For many stem cell therapies, particularly those involving novel approaches, the long-term effects and potential risks are still being investigated. It can take years or even decades to fully understand the safety profile of a treatment.

Lack of Standardization

The lack of standardized protocols for stem cell therapy can introduce variability in safety and efficacy. Different clinics and providers may use varying methods and quality controls, which can impact patient outcomes.

Experimental Treatments

Some stem cell treatments are considered experimental and may carry higher risks due to the limited data available. Patients considering these therapies should be cautious and well-informed about the potential uncertainties.

Stories of Caution

In recent years, there have been reported instances of patients seeking stem cell treatments from unregulated clinics that promise miraculous cures for a wide range of conditions. These clinics often operate without rigorous oversight or adherence to established medical standards. Patients have reported adverse events and complications following these treatments.

For example, in some cases, patients have experienced infections due to improper handling of stem cell products or unsterile conditions at the clinic. In other instances, patients have suffered from unproven treatments that didn't provide the promised benefits and may have incurred significant financial costs.

A clinic in the United States marketed stem cell treatments for conditions such as joint pain and arthritis. Several patients who received these treatments later experienced severe infections, joint damage, and complications, leading to serious health issues and the need for additional medical interventions.

Such cases underscore the importance of seeking stem cell therapy from reputable and regulated medical institutions that prioritize patient safety and adhere to established ethical and scientific guidelines.

It is essential to conduct thorough research, consult with qualified healthcare professionals, and be cautious of clinics making extravagant claims without scientific evidence. Safety should be a priority when considering stem cell treatments.

Licensing requirements and oversight of stem cell clinics can vary significantly by country and region. While there isn't a single global licensing body specifically for stem cell therapies, individuals considering stem cell treatment should check for compliance with relevant local and national regulations and licensing authorities. Here are some general guidelines:

- **FDA (Food and Drug Administration):** In the United States, the FDA regulates stem cell therapies. Patients can check if a clinic or treatment has received FDA approval or if it is part of an FDA-sanctioned clinical trial. The FDA provides information on approved stem cell therapies and clinical trials on their website.

- **EMA (European Medicines Agency):** In Europe, the EMA oversees the approval and regulation of stem cell therapies. Patients can look for EMA approval or involvement in clinical trials for European-based clinics.

- **National Health Authorities:** Many countries have their own health authorities responsible for regulating medical treatments. Patients should check with their country's health authority or equivalent agency to verify the legitimacy and licensing of stem cell clinics.

- **Medical Boards:** In some countries, healthcare professionals are required to be licensed by medical boards or councils. Patients can verify the credentials and licensing status of healthcare providers through these boards.

- **Accreditation Organizations:** Some clinics may voluntarily seek accreditation from healthcare accreditation organizations. While this is not a guarantee of treatment efficacy, it can indicate a commitment to quality and safety standards.

- **Clinical Trial Databases:** Patients interested in stem cell therapies can search for ongoing clinical trials related to their condition on databases like ClinicalTrials.gov (for the US) or the European Clinical Trials Register (for Europe). Participation in well-designed clinical trials can provide additional assurance of treatment safety and efficacy.

- **Local Regulations:** In addition to national regulations, local or state-level regulations may apply to healthcare facilities, including stem cell clinics. Patients should investigate any relevant local laws and regulations.

- **Patient Advocacy Groups:** Some patient advocacy groups maintain lists of reputable clinics and can provide guidance on where to seek treatment. They may also have information on licensed providers.

The FDA has issued multiple advisories and taken regulatory actions against clinics providing unauthorized and potentially hazardous stem cell therapies. You can find detailed information, including specific cases and adverse events, on the FDA's official website under their "Regulated Products" section.

Here are the key aspects of the FDA's guidelines and regulations related to stem cell therapies:

- **Compliance with Regulatory Pathways:** The FDA distinguishes between different types of stem cell therapies, such as minimally manipulated autologous cell therapies (lower risk) and more complex, manipulated cell products (higher risk). Stem cell products are categorized based on their level of manipulation and intended use, and they may be subject to different regulatory pathways.

- **Clinical Trials:** Stem cell therapies are typically required to undergo rigorous preclinical testing and clinical trials to establish their safety and efficacy. Clinical trials are essential for demonstrating the benefits and potential risks of a treatment.

- **Investigational New Drug (IND) Application:** For stem cell therapies that involve investigational products, sponsors may need to submit an IND application to the FDA. This application provides data on the product's safety and planned use in clinical trials.

- **Current Good Manufacturing Practices (cGMP):** The FDA requires that facilities involved in the manufacturing of stem cell products adhere to cGMP regulations to ensure product quality and consistency.

- **Informed Consent:** Patients participating in clinical trials of stem cell therapies must provide informed consent, which includes being given details about the experimental nature of the treatment, potential risks, and benefits.

- **Regulatory Enforcement:** The FDA has taken regulatory actions against clinics and providers offering unapproved and potentially risky stem cell treatments. This includes issuing warnings, conducting inspections, and taking legal actions to protect patient safety.

- **Communication and Education:** The FDA provides information and resources to educate healthcare professionals and the public about the regulation of stem cell therapies and the importance of seeking FDA-approved treatments.

- **Oversight and Monitoring:** The FDA continually monitors stem cell therapies, evaluates emerging scientific evidence, and updates its regulatory framework as needed to reflect advances in the field.

Individuals considering these procedures should be well-informed and consult with healthcare professionals who are knowledgeable about FDA regulations. Patients should also verify the legitimacy and compliance of clinics and providers offering stem cell treatments. Additionally, staying updated with the latest FDA guidelines and regulations is essential for those interested in stem cell therapies.

If you're considering treatment in the United States, keep the following points in mind:

- **Hematopoietic Stem Cell Transplants:** The FDA has approved various hematopoietic stem cell products for the treatment of conditions such as leukemia, lymphoma, and certain genetic blood disorders. These products are used in bone marrow and peripheral blood stem cell transplants.

- **Mesenchymal Stem Cell (MSC) Products:** Some MSC-based products, like alofisel (darvadstrocel), have received approval for specific conditions. For example, darvadstrocel is approved for adults with Crohn's disease who have perianal fistulas.

- **Chimeric Antigen Receptor (CAR) T-cell Therapies:** CAR T-cell therapies such as Kymriah and Yescarta, which involve genetically modifying a patient's own T-cells to target cancer cells, have been approved for certain types of leukemia and lymphoma.

- **Hematopoietic Stem Cell Cord Blood Products:** Cord blood-derived stem cell products, such as HEMACORD, have been approved for use in hematopoietic stem cell transplantation in certain clinical settings.

- **Skin Substitute Products:** Some skin substitute products, which may contain stem cells, have received FDA approval for the treatment of burns and chronic skin ulcers.

- **Bone Marrow Products:** Certain bone marrow products have received FDA approval for specific orthopedic indications, such as spinal fusion surgeries.

It's important to note that each FDA-approved stem cell product is approved for a specific medical indication and is subject to strict regulations and monitoring. The approval process involves extensive clinical trials to demonstrate safety and efficacy.

If you are exploring treatment options outside the US, keep in mind that the FDA's jurisdiction does not extend to medical treatments conducted in foreign countries. Information about overseas facilities and their stem cell products is generally limited.

It is advisable to familiarize yourself with the regulatory framework governing medical products and treatments in the specific country you are considering.

Outside the US, the International Society for Stem Cell Research (ISSCR) stands as a prominent authority within the realm of stem cell research. It offers insights, guidance, and recommendations spanning multiple facets of stem cell research and therapy, encompassing ethical deliberations and the adoption of optimal approaches. As the field is changing rapidly, it is recommended you check the ISSCR website for the latest information.

Stem Cell Treatments: What You Need to Know

ISSCR Guidelines for Stem Cell Research: These guidelines cover topics such as informed consent, patient privacy, and responsible conduct in research. These recommendations emphasize the importance of rigorous preclinical testing and adherence to regulatory requirements before initiating clinical trials. ISSCR encourages researchers and clinicians to prioritize patient safety and provide clear informed consent to participants.

- **Patient Information:** ISSCR emphasizes the importance of providing accurate and balanced information to patients considering stem cell therapies. Patients should have access to comprehensive information about the potential risks, benefits, and uncertainties associated with these treatments.

- **Unproven Stem Cell Therapies:** ISSCR has expressed concern about the proliferation of unproven and potentially unsafe stem cell therapies being offered by clinics worldwide. The organization strongly advises against the use of unproven treatments that lack scientific evidence of safety and efficacy.

- **Regulatory Oversight:** ISSCR recognizes the importance of regulatory oversight in ensuring the safety and efficacy of stem cell therapies. It encourages collaboration with regulatory agencies to establish appropriate standards and requirements for clinical trials and treatments.

- **Patient Advocacy:** ISSCR collaborates with patient advocacy groups to raise awareness about the importance of evidence-based stem cell treatments and to advocate for patient safety.

- **Educational Resources:** ISSCR provides educational resources for researchers, healthcare professionals, and the public to promote understanding and responsible engagement with stem cell research and therapies.

It's important to note that ISSCR's recommendations serve as ethical and scientific guidelines rather than legal regulations. While the organization plays a significant role in promoting best practices and ethical conduct in stem cell research and clinical applications, regulatory authorities in each country have the ultimate authority to approve and oversee stem cell therapies.

Patients and researchers can refer to ISSCR's guidelines for valuable guidance in the field of stem cell research and therapy on their website at https://www.cell.com/stem-cell-reports/fulltext/S2213-6711(23)00302-8

Other Organizations Overseeing Stem Cell Research

World Health Organization (WHO): WHO provides guidance on the use of stem cells in clinical applications and research, with a focus on ensuring safety and ethical standards.

- **European Medicines Agency (EMA):** The EMA is the regulatory agency of the European Union. It is responsible for evaluating and supervising medicinal products. They have specific regulations and guidelines related to stem cell therapies.

- **Health Canada:** Health Canada provides regulatory oversight for stem cell therapies in Canada and offers guidelines and recommendations for their safe and ethical use.

- **Japan:** Japan is renowned for its progressive approach to regulating regenerative medicine and stem cell therapies. The country introduced the Regenerative Medicine Promotion Act in 2014, establishing a framework for expedited approval of regenerative therapies. This initiative has led to several innovative treatments being approved for clinical use.

- **Australia:** Australia follows strict regulatory oversight for stem cell therapies. The Therapeutic Goods Administration (TGA) ensures that these treatments meet safety and efficacy standards. Stem cell therapies are classified as biologicals and must undergo robust evaluation and clinical trials.

- **The International Society for Cellular Therapy (ISCT):** ISCT provides guidance on various cellular therapies, including stem cell therapies, and promotes best practices in the field.

These organizations often publish reports, guidelines, and recommendations to help ensure the safe and ethical use of stem cell therapies, and their websites can be valuable resources for up-to-date information and guidance.

As we explore the regulations and legalities surrounding stem cell therapy, it becomes evident that this field is not only about scientific discovery but also about ethical considerations, patient safety, and responsible innovation. A harmonious blend of global guidelines, country-specific regulations, and vigilant patient advocacy will continue to shape the future of stem cell therapy, offering hope to patients while safeguarding their well-being.

Recommendations

- **Patient Safety:** Ensuring the safety of patients is a top priority. Stem cell therapies should undergo rigorous preclinical and clinical testing to demonstrate safety and efficacy before widespread use.

- **Ethical Considerations:** Stem cell research and therapy should be conducted in accordance with ethical principles, such as informed consent, transparency, and respect for the rights and well-being of patients.

- **Regulation and Oversight:** Regulatory agencies like the FDA, EMA, and others should oversee and regulate stem cell therapies to ensure they meet safety and quality standards.

- **Clinical Trials:** Stem cell therapies should be subject to well-designed and controlled clinical trials to assess their safety and effectiveness. Patients should be informed if they are participating in a clinical trial.

- **Transparency:** Clinics offering stem cell therapies should provide clear and accurate information about the treatment, potential risks, benefits, and alternative treatments.

- **Licensing and Accreditation:** Clinics and healthcare professionals offering stem cell therapies should be properly licensed and accredited by relevant authorities.

- **Validated Protocols:** Therapies should be based on scientifically validated protocols and methods. Clinics should not offer unproven treatments or make unsupported claims.

- **Long-Term Follow-Up:** Patients receiving stem cell therapies should undergo long-term follow-up to monitor their health and detect any adverse events or complications.

- **Patient Education:** Patients should be educated about the nature of stem cell therapies, realistic expectations, and potential risks.

- **Informed Consent:** Patients should provide informed consent after receiving comprehensive information about the therapy, including potential risks and benefits.

- **Non-Exploitation:** Patients should not be exploited, and their hopes should not be manipulated for financial gain.

We strongly support ongoing research in the field of regenerative medicine and stem cell therapies to drive progress and create treatments that are both safe and efficacious.

These recommendations strike a balance between promoting scientific progress and ensuring the safety and well-being of patients. It's important to consult the specific guidelines provided by the relevant regulatory bodies and organizations for detailed and up-to-date information.

Before undergoing any stem cell treatment, individuals should consider the following checklist of critical factors to ensure their safety and well-being:

- **Medical Examination:** To determine whether stem cell therapy is a suitable treatment choice for your particular condition, a comprehensive medical assessment from a qualified healthcare expert should be obtained.

- **Treatment Purpose:** Understand the purpose of the treatment, whether it aims to address a medical condition, enhance health, or offer potential benefits.

- **Clinic and Practitioner:** Research the clinic and healthcare practitioner extensively. Ensure they are reputable, licensed, accredited, and experienced in stem cell therapies.

- **Treatment Protocol:** Obtain detailed information about the treatment protocol, including the type of stem cells used, their source, and the method of administration.

- **Safety and Efficacy:** Inquire about the safety and efficacy of the treatment, asking for scientific evidence or clinical trial data supporting its use.

- **Risks and Complications:** Be aware of potential risks, complications, and side effects associated with the treatment. Ask for a clear explanation.

- **Patient Testimonials:** Request testimonials or case studies from previous patients who have undergone similar treatments at the clinic.

- **Regulatory Compliance:** Verify that the clinic complies with regulatory standards and guidelines set by relevant authorities in your region.

- **Informed Consent:** Ensure you provide informed consent after receiving comprehensive information about the treatment, its potential outcomes, and risks.

- **Alternative Options:** Explore alternative treatment options and consult with multiple healthcare professionals to make an informed decision.

- **Cost and Payment:** Clarify the total cost of the treatment, including any additional fees, and the payment process. Beware of high-pressure sales tactics.

- **Follow-Up Care:** Discuss post-treatment follow-up care, including monitoring and potential long-term effects, with the healthcare provider.

- **Patient Rights:** Be aware of your rights as a patient, including the right to ask questions, seek a second opinion, and decline treatment if you have concerns.

- **Treatment Location:** Consider the location of the treatment and its proximity to emergency medical facilities, in case of unforeseen complications.

- **Patient Education:** Continuously educate yourself about stem cell therapies, stay informed about regulatory changes, and seek updated information.

- **Consultation:** Schedule a consultation with the healthcare provider to discuss all aspects of the treatment, addressing any doubts or questions.

- **Legal and Ethical Considerations:** Ensure that the treatment complies with legal and ethical standards, and that the clinic operates transparently and ethically.

- **Support System:** Inform your family and friends about the treatment and consider having a support system in place during and after the procedure.

Individuals should make informed decisions and minimize potential risks associated with the treatment.

Clinical Trials

If you are considering signing up for a stem cell therapy study, consider the following points:

Understand the Nature of the Study

Know the purpose of the clinical trial, including its goals, objectives, and what researchers aim to achieve with the stem cell therapy being tested. Understand the specific stem cell product or treatment being investigated, its mode of action, and the targeted medical condition.

Informed Consent

You will be asked to provide informed consent before participating. Read the informed consent document carefully and ask questions if you have any concerns or need clarification. The informed consent form should outline the study's objectives, procedures, potential risks, benefits, and your rights as a participant.

Eligibility Criteria

Ensure that you meet the eligibility criteria for the clinical trial. These criteria may include age, medical history, the stage of your condition, and other factors.

Potential Risks and Benefits

Understand the potential risks associated with the stem cell therapy being tested. Consider factors such as side effects, complications, and any unknown risks.

Be aware of the potential benefits, but also understand that experimental therapies may not guarantee a cure or improvement.

Duration and Commitment

Know the expected duration of the trial and the level of commitment required. Clinical trials may involve multiple visits, tests, and follow-up assessments.

Regulatory Approval

Confirm whether the clinical trial has FDA approval.

Ethical and Legal Protections

Understand the ethical guidelines and legal protections in place for clinical trials. Researchers are bound by ethical principles and regulatory oversight to ensure participant safety.

Patient Support Groups

Consider joining patient advocacy or support groups related to your medical condition. These groups can provide valuable insights and support for individuals considering clinical trials.

Alternative Treatment Options

Discuss alternative treatment options with your healthcare provider. Evaluate whether participating in the clinical trial is the most suitable choice for your condition.

Review the Protocol

Carefully review the trial's protocol, which outlines the study's design, procedures, and criteria for success. This can provide a deeper understanding of what to expect.

Second Opinions

Seek a second opinion from another healthcare provider to gain additional perspectives on the trial and its potential benefits and risks.

Ask Questions

Don't hesitate to ask questions of the research team. This includes questions about the stem cell therapy, the trial's design, and any concerns you may have.

Participant Rights

Familiarize yourself with your rights as a clinical trial participant. These rights include the ability to withdraw from the trial at any time without penalty.

Long-Term Outlook

Discuss the long-term outlook with your healthcare provider. Understand how the trial may impact your ongoing treatment plan and future healthcare decisions.

Data Sharing and Publication

Inquire about the publication and sharing of study results. Researchers often publish their findings to contribute to scientific knowledge.

Communication

Maintain open and regular communication with the research team throughout the trial. Report any changes in your health or any issues you may encounter.

Patient Diary

Consider keeping a diary to record your experiences, symptoms, and any changes in your health. This can be helpful in tracking progress and identifying potential side effects.

Patient Safety Monitoring

Understand how your safety will be monitored during the trial. Clinical trials have safety protocols in place to protect participants.

Access to Post-Trial Treatment

Determine whether there is a plan in place for continued access to the stem cell therapy or other treatments after the trial concludes.

Stay Informed on Results

Stay engaged with the research team to learn about the trial's results. These results may impact your future treatment decisions.

Clinical trials are the bedrock of evidence-based medicine, serving as the crucible where innovative treatments are rigorously tested for safety and efficacy. In the context of stem cell therapy, these trials play a pivotal role in determining whether these promising interventions can truly deliver on their potential. They are a critical component of the healthcare research ecosystem, providing a structured pathway for the development and validation of novel treatments.

1. Clinical Trial Phases

- Phase 1: Safety and dosing are studied in a small group of volunteers. Side effects are identified, and medication dose or dose range is determined.

- Phase 2: The drug's efficacy is determined, and more information is gathered about side effects. The study group is larger and the dose is further defined.

- Phase 3: The study group is larger and varied, often across multiple study locations. These trials compare investigational therapy to standard treatments or a placebo to establish its efficacy, safety, and potential side effects in a real-world context.

- Phase 4: Phase 4 trials monitor a drug after it receives approval. It follows larger patient populations and tracks long-term safety and efficacy. Long-term side effects and rare events are reported.

Evidence-Based Research

Evidence-based research forms the foundation of clinical trials. It requires a meticulous and systematic approach to gathering, analyzing, and interpreting data. Stem cell therapies must be studied using this approach to ensure safety and efficacy.

2. The Dangers of Unproven Treatments

The allure of stem cell therapies has led to the emergence of clinics and providers offering unproven treatments that bypass the rigorous scrutiny of clinical trials. These unregulated interventions can pose significant risks to patients.

Consider the case of Tara, who sought stem cell therapy at a clinic promising a "miracle cure" for her multiple sclerosis. Lured by the hope of a breakthrough, she underwent the treatment, only to experience severe complications, including infection and worsening of her symptoms. Tara's experience underscores the importance of evidence-based research and the potential dangers of treatments not supported by robust clinical trial data.

3. Studies and Research Highlights

Significant progress in stem cell research has been made. The wide-ranging potential of these cells across various medical conditions is amazing. While we have discussed some of the research earlier in this book, it is important to highlight additional studies and findings that contribute to our understanding of stem cell therapy.

- **Parkinson's Disease:** A study published in *Inflammation and Regeneration* explored the use of induced pluripotent stem cells (iPSCs) to model Parkinson's disease and test potential therapies (Morizane, 2023). This research deepened our understanding of the disease and its mechanisms.

- **Cardiac Repair:** The journal *Circulation Research* demonstrated the use of stem cells in cardiac repair (Wollert & Drexler, 2005). Stem cell therapies improved heart function after heart attack.

- **Spinal Cord Injury:** A study published in *Frontiers in Cellular Neuroscience* investigated the use of stem cell-derived motor neurons to restore function in spinal cord injuries (Trawczynski et al., 2019).

As we continue to review clinical trials and research, it becomes evident that the scientific community is committed to advancing the field of stem cell therapy through rigorous investigation. The future of stem cell therapies depends on evidence-based research.

4. Challenges and Controversies

While regulations protect patients and uphold ethical standards, they are not without challenges and controversies. Stem cell therapy's rapidly evolving nature can sometimes outpace regulatory frameworks. This lag can lead to the emergence of unregulated clinics and providers offering unproven treatments.

5. Unregulated Clinics

The proliferation of unregulated clinics offering stem cell therapies poses significant risks to patients. These clinics often operate outside established regulatory frameworks, potentially exposing patients to ineffective or unsafe treatments. Ensuring that patients receive care from reputable, regulated providers is crucial for their safety.

6. Regulatory Gaps

The dynamic and innovative nature of stem cell therapy can create regulatory gaps. Addressing these gaps is essential to keep pace with scientific advancements and ensure that patients have access to safe and effective treatments.

7. Patient Advocacy and Awareness

In this intricate regulatory landscape, patient advocacy and awareness play pivotal roles. Patients and their advocates can help shape regulations, ensure compliance, and hold unscrupulous providers accountable.

One recurring theme throughout this chapter is the importance of being an informed patient. In the world of stem cell therapy, knowledge is power. By understanding the potential benefits, risks, and regulatory landscape, informed healthcare decisions can be made.

In the next chapter, we'll give you the tools and information to help you make decisions about stem cell therapy. Making the right choices requires a thoughtful and informed approach. We will outline the steps to evaluate claims, consider ethical considerations, and ultimately make decisions that align with your best interests and well-being. Stay with us as we continue this enlightening expedition into the world of stem cell therapy.

Chapter 5:
The Decision-Making Process

Making Informed Decisions

The discussion will now change to focus on the most critical decision: The decision about our own healthcare. The decision to pursue stem cell therapy is a significant one, filled with complexities, considerations, and, at times, uncertainties. To make an informed choice, we must navigate a multitude of factors, from assessing our eligibility and suitability for the therapy to finding a reputable treatment provider and addressing financial considerations.

Why Stem Cell Therapy Is Often Expensive

Before we dive into the intricacies of the decision-making process, it's essential to address a significant concern that often looms over stem cell therapy: its cost. Stem cell therapy has gained a reputation for being expensive, and this raises a fundamental question: Why is it so costly?

The expense associated with stem cell therapy can be attributed to several factors:

- **Research and Development:** Stem cell therapies undergo rigorous research and development phases, including preclinical studies and clinical trials. These stages demand substantial investments in terms of time, resources, and expertise.

- **Regulatory Compliance:** As we explored in the previous chapter, regulatory oversight is a critical aspect of stem cell therapy. Meeting regulatory standards requires extensive documentation, quality control measures, and compliance efforts.

- **Specialized Equipment and Facilities:** Stem cell therapies often necessitate specialized equipment, facilities, and highly trained personnel. The establishment and maintenance of these resources contribute to the overall cost.

- **Patient Safety:** Ensuring patient safety is paramount in stem cell therapy. Stringent measures, such as donor screening, testing, and quality control, are essential to minimize risks.

- **Quality Control:** Stem cell therapies must meet stringent quality control standards to ensure the safety and efficacy of treatments. This includes monitoring and verifying the quality of cells used.

- **Customization:** Stem cell therapies are often personalized to each patient, requiring tailored treatments and processes, which can be resource intensive.

- **Continuing Research:** Research is essential to continuously improve therapies. This commitment to research and innovation comes with associated costs.

It's important to recognize that while stem cell therapy may be costly, it also represents a significant investment in the future of medicine. These expenses are incurred in the pursuit of safer, more effective treatments that can transform lives.

Patient Eligibility and Suitability: The Maze of Possibilities

As we examine stem cell therapy, the pivotal question arises: Who is eligible and suitable for this innovative treatment? Its use is dependent on many factors, ranging from the type of disease or condition to an individual's overall health status and age.

Understanding the Complexity of Patient Eligibility

Stem cell therapy, like any medical intervention, is subject to rigorous criteria for patient eligibility. Not all individuals are suitable candidates, and a thorough evaluation is necessary to determine if this treatment aligns with the patient's needs and circumstances. Let's examine key considerations that shape patient eligibility:

Type of Disease or Condition

Stem cell therapy is not a universal cure. Its effectiveness varies based on the specific disease or condition being treated. For instance, it has shown remarkable results in treating certain blood disorders, such as leukemia, lymphoma, and multiple myeloma. In these cases, the therapy replaces malfunctioning blood cells with healthy ones derived from stem cells.

Currently, stem cell therapies are less effective or even unsuitable for conditions with complex pathologies, such as neurodegenerative diseases like Alzheimer's or Parkinson's. The intricate nature of these disorders poses challenges in directing stem cells to target the affected regions of the brain.

General Health Status

A patient's general health plays a critical role in determining eligibility. Stem cell therapy can be physically demanding, particularly in cases where it involves high-dose chemotherapy or radiation to prepare the body for stem cell infusion.

Patients with underlying health issues, weakened immune systems, or significant organ dysfunction may face increased risks during the treatment process. Their suitability for stem cell therapy must be carefully evaluated.

Age

Age is a significant factor in eligibility. While there is no universal age limit for stem cell therapy, older patients may have different considerations. For instance, elderly individuals may have age-related health concerns or reduced regenerative capacity. These factors can influence the potential risks and benefits of treatment.

Individual Factors

Beyond the broad categories of disease type, overall health, and age, individual factors further complicate the eligibility assessment. Each patient's unique medical history, genetics, and specific disease progression must be considered.

To appreciate the intricacies of patient eligibility, let's consider a few examples:

Case 1: Leukemia Treatment

A middle-aged individual is diagnosed with acute myeloid leukemia (AML), a type of blood cancer. AML is known for its aggressive nature, and stem cell therapy is a potential treatment option.

The patient's eligibility is determined through a comprehensive assessment, including tests to evaluate their overall health and the extent of leukemia. If the patient is in good health and the disease is at an early stage, they may be deemed eligible for stem cell therapy.

Case 2: Neurodegenerative Disease

An elderly patient is suffering from Parkinson's disease, a progressive neurodegenerative disorder. Stem cell therapy is under investigation as a potential treatment for this condition.

In this case, eligibility is more complex. The suitability concerns raised are age and the complexity of Parkinson's disease. A careful evaluation is required to weigh potential benefits against risks.

In the next section, we will present the process of finding reputable treatment providers—a step that can significantly impact the safety and efficacy of stem cell therapy. Making informed choices about your healthcare journey involves navigating these complex considerations, and we are here to guide you every step of the way.

Finding a Reputable Treatment Provider: Your Path to Safe and Effective Stem Cell Therapy

As you embark on the journey to explore stem cell therapy as a potential treatment option, one of the most crucial decisions you'll face is selecting a treatment provider. Your choice of a provider can significantly impact the safety, efficacy, and overall outcome of the therapy. In this section, we'll delve into the paramount importance of finding a credible and experienced medical professional and provide you with a step-by-step guide to assessing their credentials and expertise.

The Role of the Treatment Provider

Before we dive into the specifics of choosing a stem cell therapy provider, it's essential to understand the pivotal role they play in your healthcare journey. The treatment provider is not just a facilitator but a guardian of your well-being throughout the process. Here's why their role is so crucial:

- **Safety and Efficacy:** A reputable provider ensures that their stem cell therapy process adheres to the highest standards of safety and efficacy. They will use the latest research and best practices to minimize risks and maximize potential benefits.

- **Experience Matters:** Experience is often a strong indicator of a provider's ability to deliver positive outcomes. Providers who have performed numerous procedures are better equipped to handle potential complications and optimize the therapy's results.

- **Patient-Centric Approach:** Ethical stem cell therapy providers prioritize patient well-being. They will take the time to understand your unique medical history, needs, and goals, tailoring the treatment to your specific situation.

Step-by-Step Guide to Assessing a Treatment Provider

When evaluating potential stem cell therapy providers, consider these essential steps to ensure you make an informed decision:

Step 1: Verify Credentials and Specialization

Begin by verifying the provider's medical credentials and specialization. Are they licensed medical professionals with the necessary qualifications? What is the specific training and expertise? Requesting this information upfront is your first line of defense against unqualified providers.

Step 2: Evaluate Experience and Success Rates

Experience is a critical factor. Inquire about the number of stem cell procedures the provider has performed and their success rates. An experienced provider is more likely to have encountered a variety of scenarios and refined their techniques for better patient outcomes.

Step 3: Patient Reviews

Patient testimonials can offer valuable insights into a provider's track record. Reach out to former patients or look for online reviews and testimonials. However, remember that while patient experiences can be informative, individual results may vary.

Step 4: Assess Ethical Standards

Ethical standards are paramount in healthcare. Investigate whether the provider adheres to ethical guidelines and transparent practices. They should prioritize patient safety, informed consent, and clear communication throughout the treatment process.

Step 5: Ask About Research and Innovation

Inquire about the provider's involvement in ongoing research and innovation within the field of stem cell therapy. Are they current with the latest advancements? Providers who actively contribute to research are often more knowledgeable and forward-thinking.

Step 6: Red Flags to Watch For

While searching for a reputable stem cell therapy provider, keep an eye out for red flags that might indicate a lack of reliability or credibility:

- **Lack of Transparency:** Providers who are unwilling to share information about their qualifications, success rates, or procedures should raise concerns.

- **Unrealistic Claims:** Be cautious of providers who make grandiose promises or guarantee specific outcomes.

- **Pressure Sales Tactics:** Providers who pressure you into making hasty decisions or push for immediate payment may not have your best interests in mind.

- **No Informed Consent:** Ethical providers will always obtain your informed consent, explaining the potential risks, benefits, and alternatives before proceeding.

Choosing a provider is crucial. Evaluate their experience, expertise, ethical standards, and commitment to patient well-being are pivotal in ensuring safe and effective treatment. By following the steps outlined in this guide and remaining vigilant for red flags, you can navigate the path to finding a provider who aligns with your healthcare goals.

Cost

Let's break down the cost considerations:

- **Type of Stem Cell Therapy:** Different types of stem cell therapies are used to treat various medical conditions. For example, autologous stem cell therapies, which use a patient's cells, may have different costs compared to allogeneic therapies that require donor cells. Additionally, the complexity of the procedure and the number of sessions can influence the overall cost.

- **Geographic Variation:** Stem cell therapy costs vary from one country or region to another. Factors such as local healthcare infrastructure, regulatory standards, and the cost of living contribute to these variations.

- **Clinic and Provider:** The reputation, experience, and expertise of the clinic or provider can impact the cost. Established and reputable providers may charge higher fees, reflecting their experience and success rates.

- **Condition Complexity:** The underlying medical condition being treated can influence the cost. Conditions that require more extensive procedures or specialized techniques may come with higher expenses.

- **Clinical Trials:** Some patients may access stem cell therapy through participation in clinical trials. In such cases, the cost of the therapy may be covered by the trial sponsor or research institution. However, patients should be aware that clinical trials often have specific inclusion criteria, and not all participants may receive the experimental treatment.

- **Insurance Coverage:** Insurance coverage for stem cell therapy can vary. Some therapies may be considered experimental and not covered by insurance plans, while others may be covered if they are approved treatments for specific medical conditions. Patients should check with their insurance providers to understand coverage options.

- **Out-of-Pocket Fees:** Potential out-of-pocket expenses vary and can include specialist fees, laboratory tests, copays and a percentage of the total cost.

- **Consultation and Evaluation:** Patients undergo a pre-procedure work up, consisting of diagnostic tests and examinations. These pre-treatment evaluations can add to the overall cost.

- **Travel and Accommodation:** For patients seeking specialized stem cell treatments at distant centers, travel and accommodation expenses can contribute significantly to the total cost.

- **Follow-Up Care:** It's essential to consider potential follow-up care costs when planning for stem cell therapy. Patients may require additional treatments, evaluations, or medical consultations as part of their post-treatment care plan.

Insurance coverage can vary significantly based on several factors:

- **Specific Treatment:** Coverage from insurance varies depending on the type of stem cell therapy. Some treatments may be considered experimental or investigational, making them less likely to be covered.

- **Insurance Plan:** The specific insurance plan a patient holds plays a significant role. Different insurance providers may have varying policies regarding stem cell therapy coverage.

- **Healthcare System:** Insurance coverage can also be influenced by the healthcare system in a particular country. National healthcare systems, such as Medicare in the United States, may have specific guidelines regarding stem cell therapy coverage.

- **Medical Necessity:** Insurance providers will often assess the medical necessity of a treatment when determining coverage. If a treatment is deemed medically necessary and supported by clinical evidence, it may be more likely to be covered.

- **Pre-Authorization:** Some insurance plans may require pre-authorization for stem cell therapy. The insurance companies require authorization before proceeding with treatment.

- **Appeals Process:** In cases where insurance coverage is denied, patients have the option to appeal the decision. It's essential to be aware of the appeals process and be prepared to provide supporting documentation.

- **Out-of-Pocket Costs:** Even with insurance coverage, patients may still incur out-of-pocket costs, such as deductibles, co-pays, or co-insurance. These costs are significant and should be planned in advance.

Exploring Financing Options

Stem cell therapy is expensive so costs should be verified prior to completing the procedure. Here are some avenues to consider:

- **Patient Financing Programs:** Many clinics and providers offer patient financing programs that allow individuals to pay for treatment over time through manageable installments. These programs can provide financial flexibility.

- **Medical Loans:** Medical loans are a form of financing specifically designed for healthcare expenses. Patients can apply for medical loans from financial institutions or online lenders.

- **Health Savings Accounts (HSAs) and Flexible Spending Accounts (FSAs):** Individuals are allowed to set aside pre-tax dollars for eligible medical expenses. Funds from these accounts can be used to cover stem cell therapy costs.

- **Grants and Scholarships:** Some organizations offer grants or scholarships to individuals seeking stem cell therapy for specific medical conditions. Research these opportunities and their eligibility criteria.

- **Clinical Trials:** In some cases, participating in a clinical trial can provide access to stem cell therapy at reduced or no cost. The potential risks and benefits should be examined before participating in a trial.

Practical Tips for Financial Planning

Request a Detailed Cost Breakdown

Ask your treatment provider for a detailed cost breakdown that includes all potential expenses, from the procedure itself to follow-up care.

Consult Your Insurance Provider

Contact your insurance provider to discuss your policy's coverage and any pre-authorization requirements. Be prepared to provide specific details about your treatment plan.

Explore Financing Options Early

Begin exploring financing options well in advance of your planned treatment date. This allows you to make informed choices and secure financing if needed.

Consider Second Opinions

Seeking a second opinion from another healthcare professional can provide valuable insights into your treatment options and potential costs.

Advocate for Yourself

If your insurance coverage is denied, don't hesitate to advocate for yourself and pursue the appeals process. Gather all necessary documentation to support your case.

Plan for Unforeseen Expenses

Be prepared for unforeseen expenses that may arise during your treatment journey. Having a financial cushion can provide peace of mind.

While the financial considerations surrounding stem cell therapy can be daunting, careful planning and thorough research can help you make informed decisions. Understanding the costs, insurance coverage, and available financing options will empower you to navigate the financial maze and focus on your journey toward potential health improvements.

We've explored the complexities of determining the costs of treatment, deciphered the nuances of insurance coverage, and unveiled various financing options. Along the way, we've gathered practical tips to help you make informed financial decisions on your journey towards potential health improvements.

The Comprehensive Decision-Making Process for Stem Cell Therapy

As we extend our exploration of the decision-making process for stem cell therapy, we recognize the gravity of this life-altering choice. Beyond patient eligibility, reputable providers, and financial considerations, there are additional aspects to consider.

Treatment Selection

Types of Stem Cell Therapies

Stem cell therapy encompasses various approaches, including autologous, allogeneic, and induced pluripotent stem cells (iPSCs). Each type has its unique applications, benefits, and considerations. Consultation with healthcare professionals and researchers can help you identify which type aligns best with your specific medical condition.

Targeted Conditions

Stem cell therapy isn't a universal solution. It's essential to pinpoint the medical condition you are addressing. Whether it's neurodegenerative diseases like Parkinson's or autoimmune disorders like multiple sclerosis, tailoring the treatment to your condition is paramount.

Treatment Timeline

Urgency

The urgency of treatment varies depending on the medical condition. Some conditions require immediate intervention, while others allow for careful consideration and planning. Discuss with your healthcare team to determine the optimal treatment timeline.

Preparation Time

Some stem cell therapies necessitate preparation time, such as mobilizing stem cells from the bone marrow before collection. Understanding these preparatory phases is vital for timely decision-making.

Consulting Multiple Experts

Medical Specialists

Collaborate with medical specialists who have expertise in your specific condition. Seeking second or third opinions can provide valuable insights into the suitability of stem cell therapy for your case.

Stem Cell Researchers

Researchers specializing in stem cell therapy can offer comprehensive knowledge about the latest advancements, potential benefits, and ongoing clinical trials. Their expertise is invaluable in guiding your decision.

Ethical Considerations

Informed Consent

Stem cell therapy often involves experimental or innovative treatments. Ensure that you fully understand the nature of the treatment, potential risks, and expected outcomes. Informed consent is a fundamental ethical principle in healthcare decision-making.

Ethical and Legal Compliance

Verify that the chosen treatment provider adheres to ethical and legal standards. Respect for your autonomy, privacy, and dignity should be at the forefront of their practices.

Patient Advocacy

Empowering Patient Voice

Engage in open communication with your healthcare team. Your preferences, values, and goals should guide the decision-making process. Be an active advocate for your well-being.

Patient Communities

Connect with patient advocacy groups and support networks dedicated to your specific medical condition. These communities can provide valuable insights, shared experiences, and emotional support.

Post-Treatment Considerations

Follow-Up Care

After stem cell therapy, a comprehensive plan for follow-up care is essential. Discuss the post-treatment care regimen, potential complications, and long-term monitoring with your healthcare provider.

Lifestyle Adjustments

Consider how the treatment might impact your daily life. Assess potential lifestyle adjustments, including dietary changes, physical activity, and stress management, to optimize treatment outcomes.

Holistic Wellness Integration

Complementary Therapies

Explore complementary therapies that can enhance the effectiveness of stem cell treatment. These may include physical therapy, nutrition counseling, or mindfulness practices.

Mental and Emotional Health

Your well-being should be prioritized. Coping with a chronic or serious medical condition can be challenging, and seeking counseling or support when needed is essential.

Financial Safety Nets

Emergency Funds

Build an emergency fund or safety net to cover unforeseen expenses related to stem cell therapy. This financial cushion can alleviate stress during unexpected circumstances.

Regular Financial Review

Periodically review your financial plan to ensure it aligns with your treatment goals. Seek the guidance of a financial advisor when necessary.

In the intricate web of decisions surrounding stem cell therapy, the focus remains on patient-centric care. Each aspect of this comprehensive decision-making process is integral to ensuring that your journey is guided by informed choices, ethical standards, and a commitment to holistic well-being.

The next chapter outlines strategies to maximize the potential benefits of this innovative treatment, furthering your pursuit of a healthier and fulfilling life. Stay with us on this empowering journey of discovery and transformation.

Chapter 6:
Maximizing the Benefits of Stem Cell Therapy

Stem cell therapy's effectiveness hinges on many factors. In this chapter, we reveal the strategies and insights that can help you harness the full potential of stem cell therapy.

We will explore avenues such as lifestyle modifications, holistic healthcare integration, continuous health monitoring, and the power of self-education. Each of these elements plays a crucial role in not only optimizing the benefits of stem cell therapy but also in contributing to your overall well-being.

Imagine a scenario where someone embarks on a series of stem cell therapy sessions, each filled with the promise of healing and renewal. They experience remarkable improvements in their health and quality of life, their journey marked by hope and progress. And then, unexpectedly, they pause this life-altering streak, unaware of the potential consequences. As we'll soon discover in an anecdote, shared by a fellow individual seeking answers on Reddit, this abrupt halt can raise questions about the continuity of benefits and the importance of consistent engagement with stem cell therapy.

This narrative serves as a reminder that the journey of maximizing the benefits of stem cell therapy is one of commitment and continuous effort. With that notion in mind, let's begin our exploration, equipping you with the knowledge and tools needed to unlock the full potential of this innovative treatment.

Lifestyle Factors: Unlocking the Potential

Stem cell therapy's effectiveness isn't solely determined by the treatment itself; it is deeply intertwined with the lifestyle factors that surround it. In this section, we'll delve into the critical role that lifestyle choices play in achieving optimal results with stem cell therapy.

Nutrition: The Basis of Health

A well-balanced diet and proper nutrition are foundational to good health, and they become even more crucial when undergoing stem cell therapy. While there isn't a one-size-fits-all dietary plan for stem cell therapy, certain principles can guide individuals toward making nutritious choices.

Adequate nutrition provides essential building blocks for the body's repair and regeneration processes. A diet rich in vitamins, minerals, antioxidants, and protein can support tissue healing and boost the immune system, potentially enhancing the benefits of stem cell therapy.

Avoid Harmful Substances

Certain lifestyle choices, such as smoking and excessive alcohol consumption, negatively impact the body's ability to heal and recover. Smoking impairs circulation and oxygen delivery to tissues, which may hinder the effectiveness of stem cell therapy. Reducing or eliminating these harmful habits can contribute to better outcomes.

Dietary Guidelines

- Include a range of foods such as whole grains, vegetables, fruit, lean protein, healthy fats.

- Stay well-hydrated to support cellular function and overall health.

- Adequate protein intake is required for tissue repair and regeneration.

- Reducing high sodium and high sugar in foods is recommended.

- Understand that individual nutritional needs can vary significantly, so it's advisable to work with a healthcare provider or nutritionist to create a personalized dietary plan tailored to specific health goals and requirements.

Exercise and Physical Activity: Energizing the Body

Engaging in regular physical activity is another essential element of a healthy lifestyle that can complement the benefits of stem cell therapy. Exercise enhances cardiovascular fitness, promotes better circulation, strengthens muscles, and contributes to overall wellness. It may even play a role in enhancing the benefits of stem cell treatments.

However, it's vital to approach exercise with caution, especially during the recovery phase after stem cell therapy. The individual's specific needs should be considered along with age, health condition, and overall fitness level.

Exercise Guidelines

- **Consultation:** Always consult with a healthcare provider before starting an exercise program after stem cell therapy.

- **Gradual Progression:** Begin with low-intensity activities and gradually increase the intensity as tolerated.

- **Type of exercise:** Different types of exercise such as cardio, strength training, and flexibility should be used.

- **Body's Messages:** Your body will give you signs, so adjust exercise accordingly.

Stress Management

Effective stress management is also essential during the recovery process. Persistent stress can adversely impact overall health and potentially hinder the benefits of stem cell therapy. Mindfulness, meditation, deep breathing exercises, or relaxation activities are proven to be beneficial.

Implementing strategies to effectively cope with and reduce stress is crucial for overall health and well-being, as excessive stress can negatively impact both physical and mental health.

- **Meditation/Mindfulness:** Engaging in regular meditation or mindfulness practices involves focusing attention on the present moment, which can help calm the mind, promote relaxation, and build resilience against stressors.

- **Relaxation Activities:** Participating in activities such as deep breathing exercises, progressive muscle relaxation, or hobbies like gardening or painting can serve as outlets for stress relief, allowing individuals to unwind and recharge.

Fatigue Management

Fatigue can be a common side effect of stem cell therapy. Managing fatigue involves proper rest, nutrition, and engaging in activities that conserve energy. Plan for both active and rest periods.

Sleep and Rest

Adequate sleep and rest are fundamental to the body's healing processes. During sleep, the body repairs and regenerates tissues, including those affected by stem cell therapy. Maintaining adequate sleep aids in the recovery process.

Sleep Hygiene Tips

- **Consistency:** Strive for a consistent sleep routine by retiring and rising at consistent times daily.
- **Comfort:** Establish a soothing sleep atmosphere with a comfortable mattress and minimal disruptions.

- **Reduce Stimulants:** Stop caffeine and electronic gadgets in proximity to bedtime to enhance sleep quality.

- **Hydration:** Staying well-hydrated is essential for cellular function and overall health. Adequate fluid intake supports circulation, nutrient transport, and the elimination of waste products. While it's crucial to drink enough water, it's equally important not to over hydrate, as this can lead to electrolyte imbalances.

Hydration Tips

- **Balanced Intake:** Consume a variety of fluids.

- **Urine Color:** Urine color should be pale yellow, indicating proper hydration.

- **Individual Needs:** Your fluid intake changes based on factors such as climate, activity, and preference.

Social Support

- **Positive Social Connections:** Maintaining a strong support network and positive social connections can have a significant impact on overall well-being. Interacting with friends and loved ones, participating in social activities, and seeking emotional support can improve mental health and reduce stress during the stem cell therapy journey.

- **Stay Connected:** Keep in touch with friends and family, even if it's through virtual means when necessary.

- **Support Groups:** Consider joining support groups or online communities where you can share your experiences and gain valuable insights.

Holistic Healthcare

Complementary Therapies (also called Integrative Health)

Integrative health care takes a patient-centered approach, recognizing that individuals are unique and that their healthcare needs can vary widely. It blends conventional medicine with evidence-based complementary therapies to address not only physical symptoms but also the mental, emotional, and social aspects of health. This approach aims to treat the whole person, not just the disease or condition.

Enhanced Healing

Complementary therapies can promote a healing environment that supports the regeneration and integration of stem cells into damaged tissues.

Optimized Recovery

Physical therapy and rehabilitation techniques can help individuals regain strength, mobility, and function following stem cell therapy, maximizing the benefits of the treatment.

Holistic Well-Being

Integrative approaches consider the mental and emotional aspects of health, helping patients manage stress, anxiety, and depression, which can impact recovery.

Reduced Side Effects

Some complementary therapies may help alleviate side effects of stem cell therapy, such as pain, inflammation, and fatigue.

Examples of Complementary Therapies

Physical Therapy

Physical therapy focuses on improving mobility, strength, and function. It can be especially beneficial for individuals recovering from injuries or surgeries, including those undergoing stem cell therapy. Physical therapists design personalized exercise programs to address specific needs and goals.

Rehabilitation Techniques

Stem cell therapy is often used to treat musculoskeletal conditions and injuries. Integrating rehabilitation techniques, such as occupational therapy or speech therapy, can assist patients in regaining lost skills and functionality.

Nutritional Support

Proper nutrition is fundamental to health and healing. Nutritionists or dietitians can work with patients to develop dietary plans that support their recovery and overall well-being.

Mind-Body Practices

Techniques like mindfulness meditation, yoga, and tai chi can help individuals manage stress, reduce anxiety, and improve mental well-being. These practices are increasingly recognized for their role in enhancing the body's healing response.

Massage and Manual Therapies

Massage therapy and manual techniques, such as chiropractic care, can alleviate muscle tension, improve circulation, and promote relaxation.

Synergy Between Treatments

The synergy between stem cell therapy and complementary therapies lies in their combined ability to address multiple aspects of health. This collaborative approach can lead to better outcomes and a faster return to normal function.

- **Consultation:** Always consult with your healthcare provider before incorporating complementary therapies into your treatment plan.

- **Qualified Practitioners:** Seek out qualified and licensed practitioners for complementary therapies.

Personalized Treatment Plans

Every patient's journey with stem cell therapy is unique, and integrative approaches allow for highly personalized treatment plans. By considering the patient's medical history, current condition, and treatment goals, healthcare providers can tailor a comprehensive strategy that maximizes the potential benefits of stem cell therapy.

Monitoring Health and Ongoing Assessment: The Key to Successful Stem Cell Therapy

Achieving the full benefits of this innovative treatment goes beyond the initial procedure. Monitoring health and conducting ongoing assessments are critical components of ensuring the effectiveness of stem cell therapy over time.

The Importance of Regular Check-Ups

Regular health check-ups are essential in post-stem cell therapy care. They serve several crucial purposes:

- **Early Detection:** Regular monitoring allows healthcare providers to detect any changes in a patient's health status promptly. Early detection of complications or deviations from the expected course of recovery enables timely intervention and adjustments in treatment plans.

- **Assessment of Progress:** Monitoring helps assess the progress of the stem cell therapy. It allows healthcare professionals to evaluate whether the treatment is achieving its intended outcomes and whether further interventions or modifications are necessary.

- **Maintenance of Overall Health:** Beyond the specific condition targeted by stem cell therapy, regular check-ups also ensure the maintenance of overall health. They help manage other health issues and address any potential side effects or complications.

The Role of Healthcare Providers

- **Patient monitoring:** Check vital signs, conduct diagnostic tests, and assess the patient's overall well-being.

Specific Assessments

- **Blood Tests:** Blood counts and other laboratory tests are performed to monitor the patient's immune system, organ function, and overall health.

- **Imaging Studies:** Depending on the condition being treated, imaging studies like MRIs or CT scans may be used to assess the progress of tissue regeneration and detect any anomalies.

- **Physical Examinations:** Healthcare providers perform physical examinations to evaluate the patient's physical condition, including mobility, pain levels, and any signs of complications.

- **Symptom Management:** Monitoring helps in the management of symptoms and side effects. Healthcare providers can adjust medications or recommend therapies to alleviate discomfort.

Self-Monitoring and Patient Compliance

Patient involvement in their own care is paramount to the success of stem cell therapy. Patients should actively participate in self-monitoring and adhere to prescribed medication and therapy plans. This includes:

- **Self-Reporting:** Patients should promptly report any changes in their health, including new symptoms, side effects, or complications, to their healthcare providers.

- **Medication Adherence:** Adherence to prescribed medications and therapies is crucial for maintaining the effectiveness of treatment. Patients must follow their medication schedules diligently.

- **Lifestyle Modifications:** Healthcare providers may recommend lifestyle modifications, such as dietary changes or exercise routines, to support recovery and overall health. Patient compliance with these recommendations is essential.

A Collaborative Approach to Care

Effective post-stem cell therapy care is a collaborative effort between patients and their healthcare providers. It involves open communication, regular follow-ups, and a shared commitment to achieving the best possible outcomes. Patients should actively engage in their healthcare journey, ask questions, and seek clarification on any concerns.

Ensuring Successful Outcomes

The success of stem cell therapy extends beyond the initial treatment. Regular health check-ups, ongoing assessment, and patient compliance are integral components of the journey towards optimal health and well-being. By actively participating in their care and working closely with healthcare providers, patients can maximize the benefits of stem cell therapy and achieve the best possible outcomes.

Patient Empowerment and Self-Education: The Keys to Post-Stem Cell Therapy Success

One of the most potent tools at a patient's disposal is knowledge. Patient empowerment through education is instrumental in making informed decisions, adhering to treatment plans, and navigating the challenges that may arise during and after stem cell therapy.

The Power of Knowledge

Informed patients are not just passive recipients of medical care; they are active participants in their own health journey. When it comes to stem cell therapy, knowledge is a game-changer. Here's why it matters:

- **Informed Decision-Making:** Patients who understand the intricacies of their condition, the potential benefits of stem cell therapy, and the associated risks are better equipped to make informed decisions about their treatment. They can engage in meaningful discussions with their healthcare providers and actively contribute to the development of a personalized treatment plan.

- **Treatment Adherence:** Stem cell therapy often involves a series of steps, including pre-treatment preparations, the procedure itself, and post-treatment care. Patient education ensures that individuals are fully aware of what is expected of them at each stage. This knowledge promotes treatment adherence, which is crucial for successful outcomes.

- **Coping with Challenges:** Stem cell therapy can present challenges, including side effects, emotional and psychological hurdles, and uncertainties about the future. Informed patients are more resilient and better prepared to cope with these challenges. They know what to expect and can seek appropriate support when needed.

Resources for Patient Education

Empowering patients through education involves providing them with access to reliable, science-backed information. Healthcare institutions, patient support groups, and online resources are valuable outlets for acquiring knowledge. Here are some resources that can help patients on their educational journey:

- **Healthcare Institutions:** Many hospitals and medical centers offer patient education programs specific to stem cell therapy and related treatments. These programs often include informational brochures, workshops, and access to healthcare professionals who can answer questions and provide guidance.

- **Support Groups:** Joining a patient support group can be immensely beneficial. These groups provide a platform for individuals who have undergone or are undergoing stem cell therapy to share their experiences, challenges, and insights. They also offer emotional support and a sense of community.

- **Online Resources:** The internet is a vast repository of information, but it's crucial to source information from reputable websites and organizations. Websites of well-established cancer centers, medical institutions, and patient advocacy groups often offer educational materials, videos, and articles on stem cell therapy.

- **Scientific Literature:** For those who wish to delve deeper into the science of stem cell therapy, scientific literature and research papers can be valuable resources. They provide insights into the latest advancements, clinical trials, and emerging therapies.

Information Sources

While the abundance of information available online is a boon, it can also be overwhelming and, at times, unreliable. Therefore, it's essential for patients to approach information sources with discernment. Here are some tips for information sources:

- **Verify the Source:** Check the credibility of the source. Reputable institutions and recognized healthcare organizations are generally trustworthy.

- **Look for Evidence:** Seek information that is supported by scientific evidence and research. Claims that sound too good to be true without substantiating evidence should be approached with caution.

- **Consult Healthcare Providers:** When in doubt, consult healthcare providers. They can guide patients to reliable resources and address specific questions or concerns.

- **Consider Multiple Perspectives:** It's beneficial to consider information from multiple sources to gain a well-rounded understanding of a topic.

Empowerment through Education

Education is a pivotal aspect of maximizing the benefits of stem cell therapy. Informed patients are active participants in their treatment journey, equipped with the knowledge to make decisions, adhere to treatment plans, and overcome challenges. By accessing reliable resources and approaching information critically, patients can take charge of their health and well-being.

While this chapter has focused on the practical and clinical aspects of stem cell therapy, the journey is far from over. In the next chapter, we will shift our focus to the challenges facing stem cell therapy. We will explore the broader societal implications of this rapidly evolving field.

Chapter 7:
Challenges in Stem Cell Therapy

In our exploration of stem cell therapy, we've uncovered its immense potential, ethical considerations, and promising future. However, it's essential to shed light on the challenges that accompany this groundbreaking field. This chapter outlines the obstacles and hurdles that researchers, clinicians, patients, and society face as stem cell therapy becomes more widely accepted.

1. Scientific Challenges

Cell Source and Quality: Identifying and obtaining a consistent, high-quality source of stem cells for therapy remains a significant challenge. Ensuring that the cells are pure, functional, and safe is crucial to the success of treatments.

- **Immunological Compatibility:** The potential for immune rejection when using allogeneic (from a donor) stem cells is a persistent challenge. Researchers are developing strategies to minimize rejection, but it's still an obstacle.

- **Unpredictable Outcomes:** Stem cell therapy's efficacy can be unpredictable, as individual responses vary. Predicting how a specific patient will respond to treatment is challenging, making it difficult to set clear expectations.

- **Long-Term Safety:** The long-term safety is an ongoing concern. The potential for unexpected side effects or tumorigenicity (tumor formation) remains a focus of research and regulation.

2. *Ethical Issues*

Balancing scientific progress with ethical considerations is an ongoing challenge. Using embryonic tissue is controversial and raises moral concerns.

3. *Regulatory Framework*

Harmonizing regulations across different countries and regions poses challenges for both researchers and patients. Varying rules and standards complicate the global landscape of stem cell therapy.

4. *Patient Advocacy*

Ensuring patients' rights, including informed consent and transparency, can be challenging. Patient advocacy groups play a crucial role in addressing these issues.

5. *Clinical Challenges*

- **Cost:** The high cost is a definite challenge and may price many patients out of the therapy.

- **Lack of Standardization:** The lack of standardized protocols for stem cell therapy makes it challenging to compare results between studies and clinics.

- **Follow-Up and Monitoring:** Long-term monitoring and follow-up care are essential but can be challenging to implement effectively, especially for patients who receive treatment in different locations.

6. Public Perception and Misconceptions

- **Media Influence:** Media portrayal of stem cell therapy can impact public perception and contribute to misconceptions, creating challenges in managing patient expectations.

- **Stem Cell Tourism:** The rise of stem cell tourism presents ethical and safety challenges, as patients seek treatment in countries with different regulatory standards.

7. Research and Development Challenges

- **Funding:** Securing funding for stem cell research and clinical trials can be competitive and challenging, hindering the progress of promising therapies.

- **Clinical Trial Design:** Designing rigorous and well-controlled clinical trials for stem cell therapies is complex, requiring careful consideration of endpoints and controls.

8. Education and Awareness

- **Healthcare Provider Education:** Ensuring that healthcare providers are well-informed about stem cell therapy is crucial for safe and effective patient care.

- **Public Education:** Promoting accurate and accessible information about stem cell therapy to the public helps mitigate misconceptions and fosters informed decision-making.

9. Future Challenges and Unanswered Questions

- **Emerging Therapies:** As new stem cell-based therapies emerge, ensuring their safety and effectiveness while managing patient expectations will be an ongoing challenge.

- **Regenerative Medicine Integration:** Integrating stem cell therapy with other regenerative medicine approaches and existing medical practices presents challenges in standardization and collaboration.

- **Global Collaboration:** Achieving global collaboration on stem cell research and therapy standards remains a complex and evolving challenge.

10. Compare and Contrast

One of the key aspects in understanding the potential and challenges of stem cell therapy is to compare and contrast it with other related fields, such as gene therapy and traditional pharmacology. This comparative analysis sheds light on the unique qualities, advantages, and limitations of stem cell therapy, ultimately helping researchers, healthcare professionals, and patients make informed decisions about treatment options.

- **Gene Therapy:** Genes are altered in some way to treat or prevent disease. It corrects the genetic mutations involved.

- **Stem Cell Therapy:** It is not limited to genetic disorders and can be applied to a broader range of conditions, including degenerative diseases, injuries, and autoimmune disorders.

- **Comparative Advantage:** Stem cell therapy's versatility allows it to address a wider spectrum of medical conditions, while gene therapy is more focused on genetic disorders.

Traditional Pharmacology vs. Stem Cell Therapy

- **Traditional Pharmacology:** Traditional pharmacology relies on the development and administration of drugs or chemical compounds to treat diseases. These drugs often target specific molecular pathways or biochemical processes in the body.

- **Stem Cell Therapy:** Restores the function of organs or tissues, a more holistic view.

- **Comparative Advantage:** Tissue and organs are repaired. Traditional approaches mainly focus on symptom management.

Synergies and Integrative Approaches

- **Synergies:** Stem cell therapy, gene therapy, and traditional pharmacology can complement each other in certain cases. Combining therapies is being studied.

- **Integrative Approaches:** Integrative medicine involves combining conventional medical treatments with complementary therapies like stem cell therapy, physical therapy, and lifestyle modifications to provide holistic patient care.

- **Comparative Advantage:** Integrative approaches recognize the potential synergy between different treatment modalities, offering a more comprehensive and personalized treatment strategy.

By conducting comparative analyses with other medical fields, we gain insights into the distinct advantages and challenges of stem cell therapy. These insights enable healthcare professionals to tailor treatment plans to individual patient needs, optimizing the chances of successful outcomes. Additionally, ongoing research may reveal new opportunities for integration and collaboration among various therapeutic approaches, ultimately advancing the field of regenerative medicine.

Every obstacle is an opportunity for growth and improvement. Addressing these challenges requires collaboration, innovation, ethical considerations, and a commitment to advancing the field responsibly. In the face of these hurdles, we must strive to keep the promise of stem cell therapy alive, working towards a future where its potential can be harnessed for the benefit of all.

The following chapter will examine the ethical considerations, public awareness, and future directions of stem cell therapy. While challenges persist, so does the unwavering dedication of researchers, clinicians, and patients to unlock the full potential of this transformative field. Together, we explore the future of stem cell therapy with hope and resilience.

Chapter 8:
Ethical Considerations and Future Perspectives

Stem cell therapy has undoubtedly emerged as a promising frontier in modern medicine, offering unprecedented hope for those facing a myriad of medical conditions. In our journey through the world of stem cell therapy, we've explored its science, clinical applications, and practical considerations. As we embark on the final chapter of this expedition, we turn our attention to the ethical landscape that supports this rapidly evolving field.

The Ethical Nexus

Ethics in stem cell therapy extends beyond the laboratory and clinic, intertwining with societal values, patient rights, and moral imperatives. As we explore the ethical dilemmas shaping both practice and research in stem cell therapy, we will also consider the guiding principles for practitioners and researchers in their quest for healing and discovery.

A Kaleidoscope of Ethical Issues

Ethical considerations in stem cell therapy encompass a broad spectrum of topics, from patient consent and privacy, to the use of embryonic stem cells and genetic editing. Each issue raises profound questions about values, morality, and societal implications. We will illuminate these complex dilemmas and the ethical frameworks that guide responsible practice.

Ethical Issues in Stem Cell Therapy, a Complex Terrain

This section explores the multifaceted ethical issues that define the practice and research of stem cell therapy, emphasizing the delicate balance between scientific progress and ethical considerations.

Embryonic Stem Cells and Fetal Tissue: A Controversial Frontier

The controversy spurred research to find alternatives. Although the cells possess remarkable regenerative potential, their procurement raises profound moral questions. The ethical dilemma lies in the fact that obtaining embryonic stem cells often necessitates the destruction of embryos or the use of fetal tissue from terminated pregnancies.

This ethical conundrum has sparked intense debate worldwide, with varying legislative stances in different countries. Some nations have chosen to strictly regulate or even ban research involving embryonic stem cells and fetal tissue, prioritizing the sanctity of life from the moment of conception. Others adopt a more permissive approach, valuing the potential benefits of such research in advancing medical science.

Other Ethical Considerations

Genetic Modification

The genetic modification of stem cells raises ethical questions, particularly when applied to the germline (sperm or egg cells) as it can have hereditary consequences. Genetic modification techniques in stem cell therapy must be guided by regulations.

Ownership and Commercialization

Issues surrounding the ownership of stem cell lines and the commercialization of stem cell-based products are ethically complex. Balancing the pursuit of scientific knowledge and profit motives while ensuring access to therapies can be challenging.

Unproven Therapies

Many of these treatments lack scientific evidence of efficacy and safety and can potentially harm patients. Regulators and healthcare professionals must actively combat the marketing and administration of unproven therapies.

Long-Term Effects

The long-term effects are sometimes unknown, and patients should be informed about the potential risks and benefits over the course of their lifetimes.

The Ethical Principles Guiding Stem Cell Therapy

Ethical considerations surrounding stem cell therapy do not exist in isolation. They are intricately intertwined with fundamental ethical principles that guide medical practice and research.

Autonomy

Respect for patient autonomy is a cornerstone of medical ethics. Patients have the right to make informed decisions about their healthcare, including whether to undergo stem cell therapy.

Informed Consent

In clinical trials and treatments involving stem cells, obtaining informed consent from patients is crucial. The benefits versus risks and unknown issues should be clearly explained. Ensuring that patients make informed decisions about their participation is essential to respecting their autonomy.

Beneficence

Stem cell therapy is driven by the desire to benefit patients and improve their health. Practitioners must act in their patients' best interests and ensure that the potential benefits outweigh the risks. This principle underscores the importance of rigorous research and evidence-based practice.

Non-Maleficence

The principle of non-maleficence dictates that healthcare providers must do no harm to their patients. This principle aligns with the imperative to prioritize patient safety in stem cell therapy. It underscores the importance of thorough safety assessments and vigilance in monitoring patients for any adverse effects.

Justice

The principle of justice demands that the benefits and burdens of healthcare should be distributed fairly among all individuals. In the context of stem cell therapy, this principle raises questions about access and equity. Ensuring that these innovative treatments are accessible to a broad and diverse population is an ethical imperative.

Patient Safety

Stem cell therapies should prioritize patient safety. This includes rigorous preclinical testing, adherence to established safety protocols, and ongoing monitoring of patients for any adverse effects. Ensuring that therapies are safe and effective is an ethical imperative.

Equity and Access

Ethical concerns arise regarding the equitable distribution of stem cell therapies. Ensuring that these treatments are accessible to a diverse range of patients, regardless of socioeconomic status, is essential to avoid exacerbating healthcare disparities.

Transparency and Accountability

Stem cell research and therapy should be conducted with transparency and accountability. Researchers and clinicians must disclose potential conflicts of interest, accurately report results, and adhere to ethical guidelines and regulations.

International Collaboration

Ethical considerations in stem cell therapy often transcend national boundaries. International collaboration and adherence to global ethical standards are essential to ensure responsible and ethical practices.

Guarding Against Exploitation

The prospect of hope and healing that stem cell therapy offers can lead to patient vulnerability. Patients grappling with debilitating conditions may be susceptible to exploitation by unscrupulous clinics and providers promising miraculous cures.

The phenomenon of "stem cell tourism" highlights the ethical concerns surrounding the marketing of unproven treatments.

Transparency and informed consent emerge as essential safeguards against such exploitation. Patients must receive clear, accurate, and unbiased information about the risks, benefits, and uncertainties associated with stem cell therapy. Informed consent ensures that individuals make decisions about their healthcare based on a genuine understanding of the treatment and its implications.

An Ethical Landscape

The ethical landscape of stem cell therapy requires balancing the imperatives of scientific progress and the ethical considerations that support the practice and research of regenerative medicine. Each ethical issue presents a complex interplay of values, principles, and societal perspectives.

Public Perception: Myths and Realities

Stem cell therapy stands as a promising frontier, offering the potential for revolutionary treatments and life-altering interventions. However, beyond the laboratory and clinical settings, lies a complex public perception that is shaped by a multitude of factors, including media representation, patient advocacy groups, and individual understanding. This section examines public perception, unraveling both misconceptions and accurate understandings of stem cell therapy.

Misconceptions and Myths

Public perception of stem cell therapy is often clouded by misconceptions and myths that have persisted over the years. It is crucial to identify and address these misunderstandings to encourage a better and more knowledgeable conversation around this innovative medical field.

Stem Cells Can Cure Everything

One prevalent misconception is the belief that stem cells possess a universal power, capable of curing any ailment or disease. While stem cells indeed hold tremendous therapeutic potential, their applications are highly specialized and vary depending on the condition. Stem cell therapy is not a cure-all.

Stem Cell Therapy Is Always Risk-Free

Another common myth is the perception that stem cell therapy is entirely risk-free. Stem cell treatments have shown safety so far, but they still have risks and side effects. As with any medical intervention, careful evaluation and monitoring are essential.

Stem Cell Therapy Is Only for the Wealthy

Stem cell therapy's cost can be a barrier for many individuals, leading to the misconception that it is exclusively accessible to the wealthy. However, this perception overlooks the evolving landscape of healthcare financing and insurance coverage, which may provide options for a broader range of patients.

All Stem Cell Clinics Are Equal

Not all stem cell clinics adhere to the same rigorous standards and ethical guidelines. The perception that all clinics offer identical services can lead to unregulated and potentially unsafe treatments. Patients must exercise caution and choose reputable, regulated providers.

Stem Cells Are Derived from Embryos

A common misconception surrounding stem cell therapy is the belief that all stem cells are derived from embryos. As previously discussed, other tissues are being used in place of embryonic tissue.

Media Representation and Its Influence

Media plays a significant role in shaping public perception, and its portrayal of stem cell therapy can be both informative and influential. News articles, documentaries, and online content have the power to disseminate accurate information or perpetuate misconceptions.

Media representation often highlights breakthroughs and promising results in stem cell research. While this can inspire hope and optimism, it may also inadvertently create unrealistic expectations among the public. It is essential for media outlets to strike a balance between reporting scientific advancements and providing context about the complexities and limitations of stem cell therapy.

Media outlets sometimes frame regenerative medicine within sensationalized narratives, potentially contributing to misconceptions. Responsible reporting and science communication are crucial in fostering a more accurate understanding of stem cell therapy.

The Role of Patient Advocacy Groups and Public Education

Patient advocacy groups play a pivotal role in shaping public perception and understanding of stem cell therapy. These organizations are often formed by individuals who have a personal stake in stem cell research and therapy due to their own medical conditions or those of their loved ones.

Patient advocacy groups serve as valuable sources of information and support for individuals seeking information about stem cell therapy. They can provide firsthand accounts of experiences, offer guidance on accessing treatments, and raise awareness about the ethical and practical considerations surrounding stem cell therapy.

Public education initiatives led by these groups can help dispel myths and provide accurate information to those in need. Furthermore, they often advocate for policies that promote ethical research and access to stem cell therapies.

Public perception of stem cell therapy is shaped by a complex interplay of factors, including misconceptions, media representation, and the efforts of patient advocacy groups. Addressing misconceptions, promoting responsible media coverage, and fostering public education are essential steps in cultivating a more informed and balanced understanding of stem cell therapy. As we move forward, it is imperative to continue engaging in open and transparent dialogues that align with the ethical principles and realities of this rapidly evolving field.

Trends and Future Directions

Emerging trends and future directions offer a glimpse into the potential on the horizon.

Recent Studies

Researchers at Memorial Sloan Kettering Cancer Center found that disrupting a single gene called SUV39H1 gave CAR T-cells more staying power to fight cancer (Stallard, 2023). This approach improved CAR T-cell effectiveness against multiple cancers in mice and could potentially help CAR T-cells maintain their function, which could expand the pool of patients eligible for this treatment.

A study published in the journal *Frontiers in Public Health* found that stem cell therapy is being used to treat COVID-19 worldwide and the lives of many critically ill patients have been saved (Zhang et al., 2022).

Innovative Techniques

CRISPR gene editing has emerged as a revolutionary tool in the field of stem cell therapy. This innovative technology allows scientists to precisely modify the genetic code of stem cells, opening remarkable possibilities for personalized and targeted treatments. Using CRISPR, genetic mutations causing diseases can be corrected. The precision and versatility of CRISPR make it a game-changer in regenerative medicine, paving the way for the development of highly effective and customized stem cell-based treatments for a wide range of conditions, from genetic disorders to degenerative diseases. As CRISPR-based approaches continue to evolve, they hold the potential to revolutionize the landscape of stem cell therapy and bring newfound hope to patients seeking innovative and tailored medical solutions.

Exosome-based therapies represent an exciting frontier in stem cell research and regenerative medicine. Exosomes are tiny vesicles released by stem cells that contain a payload of bioactive molecules, including proteins, RNAs, and growth factors. These exosomes play a pivotal role in intercellular communication and are known for their regenerative and immunomodulatory properties. In the context of therapy, exosomes can be isolated from stem cells and used to deliver therapeutic cargo to target tissues. This approach holds immense promise for a variety of applications, such as tissue repair, reducing inflammation, and even potentially treating neurodegenerative diseases and autoimmune conditions. Exosome-based therapies offer the advantage of being less invasive and potentially safer than direct stem cell transplantation, making them a compelling avenue for the development of novel treatments that harness the body's own healing mechanisms. As research in this field progresses, exosome-based therapies are poised to make a significant impact on the future of regenerative medicine.

Immunotherapy combined with stem cells has shown efficacy in treating certain diseases, especially cancer. Stem cells can be harnessed to enhance the body's immune response, a concept known as immunomodulatory therapy. By engineering or modifying stem cells, researchers can create potent immunotherapies that target cancer cells more effectively. Stem cell-derived immunotherapies have the potential to precisely recognize and destroy cancer cells, while sparing healthy tissue, minimizing side effects, and improving the overall success of cancer treatments. This convergence of stem cell therapy and immunotherapy exemplifies the transformative power of multidisciplinary approaches, offering new hope and innovative solutions for patients facing challenging diseases like cancer. As research in this field progresses, the synergy between stem cells and immunotherapy holds immense promise for the future of cancer treatment and other immune-related disorders.

The Confluence of AI and Stem Cell Research

AI has revolutionized data analysis, enabling researchers to process vast datasets quickly and uncover patterns that might have gone unnoticed.

Machine learning algorithms can predict the behavior of stem cells, guide differentiation protocols, and identify optimal conditions for cell growth. AI-driven approaches enhance the efficiency of drug screening and toxicity testing, reducing the time and cost of bringing new therapies to market.

AI assists in automating the labor-intensive task of quality control during the production of stem cell-based therapies, ensuring product consistency and safety. As AI continues to advance, its synergy with stem cell research holds the promise of accelerating breakthroughs in regenerative medicine.

Towards Organ Regeneration

Tissue Engineering: Stem cell research is contributing to advances in tissue engineering, where artificial organs and tissues can be created using a patient's own cells. This has the potential to revolutionize organ transplantation and address the shortage of donor organs.

One notable advancement is the development of bioengineered organs or tissues using a combination of stem cells, biomaterials, and 3D printing technology. These techniques aim to create functional replacements for organs. While this field is still in its infancy, it offers hope for addressing the global shortage of organ donors.

Recent studies have shown promising results in animal models, suggesting that regenerating nerve tissue may become a reality in the not-so-distant future.

Curing Currently Incurable Diseases

Curing currently incurable diseases holds significant promise but here are some key points to consider:

- **Diabetes:** Researchers are investigating the use of stem cells, particularly pancreatic islet cells, for the treatment of diabetes. These cells have the potential to replace damaged insulin-producing cells in the pancreas.

- **Cancer:** Bone marrow transplants (hematopoietic stem cell transplants) have been used for many years in the treatment of blood-related cancers like leukemia and lymphoma. As for solid tumor cancers, research holds both promise and challenges. Here are some key points about the possibility of treating solid cancers with stem cells:

- **Tumor Microenvironment:** Solid tumors consist not only of cancer cells but also of a complex microenvironment that includes blood vessels, immune cells, and supporting tissues. This microenvironment can influence tumor growth and treatment response.

- **Stem Cells and Regeneration:** Because stem cells can even become cells found in solid tumors, they have been investigated to target and potentially regenerate or repair damaged tissues within tumors.

Researchers are exploring several approaches to using stem cells in cancer treatment, including:

Targeted Delivery

Stem cells can be engineered to carry therapeutic agents directly to tumor sites. This targeted delivery approach aims to minimize damage to healthy tissues while delivering treatments to cancer cells.

Immunotherapy

Certain types of immune cells, such as T cells, can be genetically modified or derived from stem cells to enhance their ability to recognize and attack cancer cells.

Tissue Engineering

Used for research, drug development and personalized medicine.

Challenges and Risks

While stem cell-based cancer therapies hold promise, there are significant challenges and risks to consider:

Tumor Heterogeneity

Solid tumors are often heterogeneous, meaning they consist of diverse cell populations. Targeting all cancer cells effectively can be challenging.

Safety Concerns

Unintended consequences are possible, such as increasing tumor growth, or side effects.

Immune Response

Immune rejection of stem cells or their products can be a concern in clinical applications.

Regulatory Approval

Developing and gaining regulatory approval for stem cell-based cancer therapies is a complex process that requires rigorous preclinical and clinical testing.

Clinical Trials

Some trials are ongoing to investigate these approaches in various cancer types.

Combination Therapies

Stem cell-based therapies are often explored in combination with other conventional cancer treatments, such as chemotherapy, radiation therapy, and immunotherapy, to enhance treatment outcomes.

While there is promise in using stem cells for targeted delivery and immunotherapy, significant research and clinical trials are needed to fully understand their potential and address safety concerns. Patients can consider participating in clinical trials when appropriate to access the latest advances in cancer treatment.

Global Efforts

Stem cell research and therapy are global endeavors, with collaboration among researchers, institutions, and countries. This collaboration accelerates progress and the sharing of knowledge.

Case Studies

Kristin Comella

Kristin Comella is often referred to as the "Queen of Stem Cells." She has been a prominent advocate for the use of stem cell therapy and regenerative medicine. Comella's own personal experience with stem cell therapy following a skiing accident fueled her passion for promoting the treatment's benefits. She has since become a key figure in the field and has worked on numerous research and clinical projects (Gellman, 2021).

Gordon McConnell

Gordon McConnell, a retired firefighter, underwent stem cell therapy to treat his chronic obstructive pulmonary disease (COPD). After the treatment, he reported significant improvements in his lung function and overall quality of life. His story highlights the potential of stem cell therapy for respiratory conditions.

Laura Dominguez

Laura Dominguez, a young woman with type 1 diabetes, participated in a clinical trial exploring the use of stem cells to treat diabetes. The trial aimed to use stem cells to regenerate insulin-producing cells in the pancreas. While the research is ongoing, Laura's willingness to participate showcases the hope that stem cell therapy offers to individuals with chronic conditions.

Jack Crick

He was cured of X-linked severe combined immunodeficiency (X-SCID) by receiving a stem cell transplant from his brother's umbilical cord blood when he was six months old. He is now a healthy teenager who enjoys sports and music (German Stem Cell Network, 2020).

The Berlin Patient

He was the first person to be cured of both HIV and leukemia by receiving a stem cell transplant from a donor who had a rare genetic mutation that made him resistant to HIV. He has been free of the virus for over 10 years (Francis Crick Institute, 2023).

Hassan

He was a "butterfly child" who suffered from a severe form of epidermolysis bullosa, a genetic skin disorder that causes blisters and wounds. He received a stem cell therapy that used genetically modified skin cells to replace his damaged skin. He now has a normal life expectancy and improved quality of life (German Stem Cell Network, 2020).

Carol Mulumba

She was diagnosed with sickle cell anemia at three weeks old. She received a stem cell transplant from her sibling's cord blood after chemotherapy. She was cured of sickle cell disease and has no signs of complications (German Stem Cell Network, 2020).

The Future in Veterinary Medicine

Stem cell therapy is being used in animals for several reasons:

Treatment of Injuries and Diseases

Stem cell therapy can effectively treat various injuries and diseases in animals. It has shown promise in addressing conditions like osteoarthritis, tendon and ligament injuries, spinal cord injuries, and certain systemic diseases.

Pain Management

Stem cell therapy can provide pain relief and improve the quality of life for animals suffering from chronic pain conditions. This is particularly beneficial for older pets with arthritis or degenerative joint diseases.

Reduced Need for Medications

In some cases, stem cell therapy can reduce the reliance on long-term medications and their potential side effects. This can be advantageous for animals with conditions that require ongoing medication management.

Enhanced Healing

Stem cells have regenerative properties that can accelerate tissue healing and repair. This can be crucial in cases of traumatic injuries or surgeries.

Improved Mobility

Animals with musculoskeletal conditions or injuries often experience improved mobility and joint function after stem cell therapy, allowing them to lead more active lives.

Minimized Side Effects

Stem cell therapy, especially when using the animal's own cells (autologous therapy), generally has minimal side effects or risks, making it a safer option for certain conditions.

Alternative to Surgery

In some instances, stem cell therapy can provide an alternative to surgical interventions, reducing the invasiveness and potential complications associated with surgery.

Research and Advancements

The use of stem cell therapy in animals contributes to ongoing research and advancements in both veterinary and human medicine. Findings in animal studies can inform human clinical trials and vice versa.

Complementary Treatments

Stem cell therapy can complement traditional veterinary treatments, such as physical therapy, medications, and surgery, to improve overall outcomes for animals.

Improved Quality of Life

Stem cell therapy can enhance the overall quality of life for animals by alleviating pain, improving mobility, and reducing the progression of certain diseases.

Veterinary Medicine Advancements

The integration of stem cell therapy into veterinary medicine reflects the field's commitment to staying at the forefront of medical advancements and providing innovative solutions for animal health.

While stem cell therapy offers numerous benefits for animals, it may not be suitable for all conditions or all individual cases. Veterinarians carefully assess each animal's condition and medical history to determine the appropriateness of stem cell therapy and create customized treatment plans. As research in veterinary regenerative medicine continues to grow, the range of conditions that can be treated with stem cell therapy is likely to expand, benefiting a wider spectrum of animals.

The Ever-Advancing Frontier

With stem cell therapy, scientific understanding is dynamic and continually evolving. What was once deemed impossible may become achievable through diligent research and innovative technologies. With the future of stem cell therapy, it is crucial to maintain an open mind, embrace emerging trends, and remain at the forefront of scientific progress.

The convergence of AI and stem cell research, the pursuit of organ regeneration, and the quest to cure currently incurable diseases herald an era of unprecedented possibilities. Stem cell therapy, once a realm of speculation, is gradually transitioning into an arena where hope meets reality. In this ever-advancing frontier, the potential for transformative breakthroughs in healthcare and regenerative medicine awaits those who dare to explore its depths.

Ethical Considerations Shaping the Future

We have explored the ethical principles that guide medical practice and research, emphasizing autonomy, beneficence, non-maleficence, and justice. These principles direct the ethical compass of stem cell therapy, ensuring that patient welfare and the greater good remain at the forefront.

We highlighted the paramount importance of transparency and informed consent in mitigating the risk of exploiting patients' hopes. Stem cell therapy offers tremendous promise, but ethical considerations must always be woven into the fabric of its practice.

Public perception was next. We acknowledged the misconceptions and accurate understandings that shape the public's view of stem cell therapy. Media representation, with its profound influence, revealed its power to mold perceptions and instill hope or skepticism.

We also celebrated the role of patient advocacy groups and public education in fostering a deeper understanding of stem cell research and therapy. These voices amplify awareness and empower individuals to make informed decisions about their healthcare.

We then gazed into the horizon of emerging trends and future directions in stem cell therapy. The confluence of artificial intelligence and stem cell research emerged as a game-changer, promising to expedite discoveries and treatments. The potential for organ regeneration and cures for currently incurable diseases ignited hope for countless patients.

Through case studies and ongoing research, we witnessed the tangible impact of these emerging trends. Vision restoration, cardiac regeneration, and patient-specific treatments showcased the transformative potential of stem cell therapy.

The Road Ahead

It is essential to acknowledge that our voyage is far from over. Stem cell therapy remains a dynamic field where scientific understanding evolves, and the boundaries of what is possible continue to expand.

In the final part of the book, we will gather the threads of knowledge we've woven throughout this journey. We'll summarize key takeaways, reiterate the importance of making informed decisions, and offer concluding thoughts and encouragement. The road ahead may be winding, but with knowledge, ethics, and a steadfast commitment to progress, we embark on the next leg of our expedition, ready to shape the future of stem cell therapy.

Conclusion

Reflections on the Journey

It is time to review where we are with stem cell therapy. We won't revisit every corner of this journey, but we will distill the essence of our exploration into a few key takeaways. So, let's conclude the last leg of our voyage, reinforced by the knowledge and inspiration we've gathered.

Key Takeaway 1: A Glimpse into the Future

Through the pages of this book, we've ventured into the future of medicine—a future where diseases are not insurmountable barriers but mere hurdles on the path to recovery. Stem cell therapy has revealed numerous possibilities, offering the hope of treatments that can transform lives, restore health, and alleviate suffering. We've explored the frontiers of regenerative medicine and glimpsed the potential for organ regeneration, vision restoration, and personalized therapies. The future holds the promise of cures for once-incurable conditions, and it's a future filled with hope.

Key Takeaway 2: Informed Decision-Making

One resounding message throughout our journey has been the paramount importance of informed decision-making. Whether you're a patient seeking treatment, a healthcare professional who is guiding patients, or simply someone curious about the science of stem cells, knowledge is your most powerful ally.

Understanding the details of stem cell therapy, from its scientific background to the regulatory landscape, empowers you to make choices that align with your best interests.

We have examined eligibility and suitability, explored the significance of finding reputable treatment providers, outlined the financial considerations and insurance coverage, and discussed the critical role of patient advocacy and self-education. Armed with this knowledge, you are better equipped to make informed decisions that can impact lives positively.

Key Takeaway 3: Ethical Considerations Matter

Ethics, an ever-present guiding star, has illuminated our path. We've recognized the delicate balancing act between scientific progress and ethical considerations. We've explored the power of public perception, media influence, and the role of patient advocacy in shaping the ethical landscape of stem cell therapy. These ethical considerations are not abstract concepts but the moral framework that ensures treatments remain grounded in principles of beneficence, non-maleficence, and justice.

Key Takeaway 4: The Future Awaits

We stand before a future brimming with possibilities. Stem cell therapy continues to evolve, driven by emerging trends and groundbreaking research. Artificial intelligence, regenerative medicine, and personalized treatments beckon us toward a brighter tomorrow.

Patient empowerment and self-education are the keys to unlocking the full potential of stem cell therapy. By staying informed, advocating for ethical practices, and participating in the ongoing advancements of this field, we become active contributors to the future of medicine.

A Success Story: The Road Ahead

Every journey deserves a success story, and this one is no exception. The success story we carry with us is one of hope, resilience, and the relentless pursuit of better healthcare. It is the story of patients who found renewed health and vitality through stem cell therapy, of healthcare professionals who dedicated their lives to improving patient outcomes, and of researchers who illuminated the path toward groundbreaking discoveries.

The success story is not just about looking back at how far we've come; it's about looking ahead to where we can go. The road ahead may be challenging, but it's also leading to a destination brimming with potential. Whether you're a patient, a healthcare professional, or someone curious about the science of stem cells, we can all strive for a future where diseases are mere setbacks, not dead ends. Together, through informed decisions and scientific advancements, we can help shape the future of medicine.

A Call to Action: Your Voice Matters

Before we bid farewell to this journey, we have one last request—a call to action. Your voice matters in the future of stem cell therapy. If this journey has inspired you, if it has armed you with knowledge, and if it has kindled a passion for the possibilities of regenerative medicine, then we ask you to share your insights and experiences by leaving a review.

A review helps share this knowledge with others, and join the chorus of voices advocating for ethical, informed, and innovative healthcare. Our collective efforts can propel stem cell therapy toward new horizons, where more patients can experience the life-changing benefits it offers.

In closing, we thank you for accompanying us on this voyage. From the depths of science to the heights of hope, we've explored the world of stem cell therapy together. As you continue your journey, may you carry the torch of knowledge, the flame of ethics, and the beacon of hope to illuminate the path toward a brighter future in medicine.

Glossary

Adult Stem Cell: an undifferentiated cell found in the body that can divide to replace cells and repair tissues.

Allogeneic: Stem cells derived from a donor's body and used for another person's treatment.

Autologous: Stem cells derived from the patient's own body and used for their own treatment.

Blood: Blood collected from the umbilical cord and placenta after childbirth, a potential source of hematopoietic stem cells.

Clinical Trial: A type of research that studies new tests and treatments and evaluates their effects on human health outcomes. Clinical trials involve human participants who are assigned to different interventions, such as drugs, devices, or procedures, and are monitored for the changes in their health conditions.

Differentiation: The process by which cells or tissues change from relatively generalized to specialized cell types with specific functions when mature.

Embryonic Stem Cell: A cell derived from the early stages of an embryo which can differentiate into any type of body cell. Embryonic stem cells can become any cell type in the body.

Ethical Considerations: Principles and guidelines that researchers and other professionals must follow to ensure that their work is ethical and responsible.

Graft-versus-Host Disease (GVHD): A complication that can occur after stem cell transplantation when the donor's immune cells attack the recipient's tissues.

Hematopoietic Stem Cell: A cell that can produce blood cells, such as red blood cells, white blood cells, and platelets. It is also able to self-renew, which means it can make more copies of itself. Hematopoietic stem cells are important for blood formation, immunity, and tissue repair.

Immunosuppression: The suppression of the immune system's activity, often necessary after stem cell transplantation to prevent rejection.

Induced Pluripotent Stem Cell (iPSC): A type of pluripotent stem cell that can be generated directly from a somatic cell, such as a skin or blood cell, by reprogramming it back into an embryonic-like state. They can differentiate into any type of cell in the body making them a valuable tool for research and medical purposes.

Informed Consent: The process of providing detailed information to patients about the risks, benefits, and alternatives of a medical procedure, ensuring they make a knowledgeable decision.

Mesenchymal Stem Cell (MSC): Cells that can differentiate into various cell types, such as bone, cartilage, muscle, and fat cells. They modulate immune responses and promote tissue repair. They come from bone marrow, cord blood, adipose tissue and dental pulp.

Multipotent: Cells that can develop into more than one cell type, but are more limited than pluripotent cells. Adult stem cells and cord blood stem cells are considered multipotent.

Pluripotent: The ability of a cell to differentiate into many cell types except the placenta. A cell is undifferentiated but capable of developing into different types of mature cells of the body.

Regenerative Medicine: A branch of medicine that aims to restore or replace damaged or diseased cells, tissues, or organs using various methods, such as stem cell therapy, tissue engineering, and biomaterials. Regenerative medicine can potentially treat many conditions, such as diabetes, heart disease, brain injury, and skin wounds.

Stem Cell: A type of cell that can divide and produce more stem cells or different types of specialized cells, such as blood cells, nerve cells, or muscle cells. They are the source of all the cells that make up the tissues and organs of animals and plants.

Tissue Engineering: A field of biomedical engineering that aims to create artificial tissues that can replace or repair damaged ones in the human body.

References

Aliouche, H. (2023, May 18). *History of stem cells.* https://www.news-medical.net/life-sciences/History-of-Stem-Cells.aspx

Anthony Nolan. (2023, November 11). *Diet after a stem cell transplant.* https://www.anthonynolan.org/patients-and-families/recovering-a-stem-cell-transplant/diet-after-a-stem-cell-transplant

Biobanking.com. (2022, June 9). *Stem cell banking: Current trends, emerging issues and challenges.* https://www.biobanking.com/stem-cell-banking-current-trends-benefits-emerging-issues-and-challenges/

Braunsteiner, N., Vickers, E., & Shparberg, R. (2018, March). Psychological issues for patients undergoing stem cell therapy and regenerative medicine. *Open Journal of Regenerative Medicine, 7(2).* https://www.scirp.org/journal/paperinformation.aspx?paperid=86941

Cancer.net. (2022, July). *The importance of follow-up care.* https://www.cancer.net/survivorship/follow-care-after-cancer-treatment/importance-follow-care

Chauhan, R. (2022, September 26). *15 best stem cell treatment in the world.* Clinic Spots. https://www.clinicspots.com/blog/best-stem-cell-therapy-hospitals-in-the-world

City of Hope. (2022, April 21). *Allogeneic stem cell transplant.* https://www.cancercenter.com/treatment-options/hematologic-oncology/allogeneic-stem-cell-transplant

Cona, L. (2024, February 2). *Stem cell therapy for liver disease: Overview, benefits & risks (2024).* DVCStem. https://www.dvcstem.com/post/can-stem-cells-treat-liver-disease

Cona, L. (2023, April 28). *Stem cell therapy for neurological disorders.* DCCStem. https://www.dvcstem.com/post/stem-cell-therapy-for-neurological-disorders

Cona, L. (2024, February 21). *Stem cell therapy: Overview, benefits & risks (2024).* DVCStem. https://www.dvcstem.com/post/stem-cell-therapy

Dagnino, A., Chagastelles, P., Medeiros, R., Estrazulas, M., Kist, L., Bogo, M., Weber, J., Campos, M., & Silva, J. (2020, November 25). Neural regenerative potential of stem cells derived from the tooth apical papilla. *Stem Cells & Development, 29(23).* https://www.liebertpub.com/doi/10.1089/scd.2020.01

Falanga, V. (2012, June). Stem cells in tissue repair and regeneration. *Journal of Investigative Dermatology, 132(6)*. https://www.ncbi.nlm.nih.gov/pmc/articles/PMC4084617/

Fuloria, S., Jain, A., Singh, S., Hazarika, I., Salile, S., & Fuloria, N.K. (2021). Regenerative potential of stem cells derived from human exfoliated deciduous (SHED) teeth during engineering of human body tissues. *Current Stem Cell Research & Therapy. 16(5)*, 507–517.https://pubmed.ncbi.nlm.nih.gov/33390148/

Gellman, L. (2021, July 1). *How fringe stem cell treatments won allies on the far right.* Wired. https://www.wired.com/story/stem-cell-treatment-far-right/

Hassan, A., Hassan, G., & Rasool, Z. (2009). Role of stem cells in treatment of neurological disorders. *International Journal of Health Sciences (Qassim), 3(2)*, 227–33. https://www.ncbi.nlm.nih.gov/pmc/articles/PMC3068820/

Henderson, E. (2022, November 10). *Research reveals why stem cell transplants are so successful in MS patients.* News Medical. https://www.news-medical.net/news/20221110/Research-reveals-why-stem-cell-transplants-are-so-successful-in-MS-patients.aspx

Henderson, E. (2023, April 17). *Combination treatment could improve stem cell transplantation process for multiple myeloma patients.* News Medical. https://www.news-medical.net/news/20230417/Combination-treatment-could-improve-stem-cell-transplantation-process-for-multiple-myeloma-patients.aspx

Hildreth, C. (2022, December 21). *Top 8 stem cell quotes of all-time.* Bioinformant. https://bioinformant.com/stem-cell-quotes/

Jones, O., & McCurdy, D. (2022, May 9). Cell based treatment of autoimmune diseases in children. *Frontiers in Pediatrics, 10.* https://www.frontiersin.org/articles/10.3389/fped.2022.855260/full

JoshSN. (2013). *I recently had a stem cell transplant to treat an autoimmune disorder, ask me anything.* Reddit. https://www.reddit.com/r/IAmA/comments/1d0mkq/i_recently_had_a_stem_cell_transplant_to_treat_an/

Kania-Richmond, A., & Metcalfe, A. (2017). Integrative health care – What are the relevant health outcomes from a practice perspective? A survey. *BMC Complementary Medicine & Therapies, 17.*

https://bmccomplementmedtherapies.biomedcentral.com/articles/10.1186/s12906-017-2041-4

Knoepfler, P. (2023, June 15). *Stem cell therapy cost in 2024: data & analysis*. The Niche. https://ipscell.com/2023/06/stem-cell-therapy-cost-in-2023-new-data/

Lindvall, O., & Kokaia, Z. (2006, June 29). Stem cells for the treatment of neurological disorders. *Nature, 441(7097)*, 1094–6. https://pubmed.ncbi.nlm.nih.gov/16810245/

Liu, D., Cheng, F., & Pan, S. (2020). Stem cells: A potential treatment option for kidney diseases. *Stem Cell Research & Therapy 11(249)*. https://stemcellres.biomedcentral.com/articles/10.1186/s13287-020-01751-2

Lund University. (2023, February 28). *First patient receives milestone stem cell-based transplant for Parkinson's disease.* https://www.lunduniversity.lu.se/article/first-patient-receives-milestone-stem-cell-based-transplant-parkinsons-disease

Malakar, D., Malik, H., Kumar, D., Saini, S., Sharma, V., Fatima, S., Bajwa, K., & Kumar, S. (2021). Chapter 3: Stem cells: a potential regenerative medicine for treatment of diseases. In S. Mondal & R. Singh (Eds.), *Advances in Animal Genomics,* (pp 33–48). Academic

Press. https://www.sciencedirect.com/science/article/abs/pii/B9780128205952000035

Maniar, H., Tawari, A., Suk, M., & Horwitz, D. (2015, November 9). The current role of stem cells in orthopaedic surgery. *Malaysian Orthopaedic Journal, 9(3)*, 1–7. https://www.ncbi.nlm.nih.gov/pmc/articles/PMC5393127/

Mayo Clinic Staff. (2024, March 23). *Stem cells: What they are and what they do*. Mayo Clinic. https://www.mayoclinic.org/tests-procedures/bone-marrow-transplant/in-depth/stem-cells/art-20048117

Medical Tourism Magazine. (n.d.). *Patient success stories: Stem cell therapy transformations in Mexico*. https://www.magazine.medicaltourism.com/article/patient-success-stories-stem-cell-therapy-transformations-in-mexico

Mohammedsaleh, Z. (2022). The use of patient-specific stem cells in different autoimmune diseases. *Saudi Journal of Biological Sciences, 29(5)*, 3338–3346. https://www.sciencedirect.com/science/article/pii/S1319562X22000857

Morizane, A. (2023). Cell therapy for Parkinson's disease with induced pluripotent stem cells. *Inflammation and Regeneration,* *43(16).* https://inflammregen.biomedcentral.com/articles/10.1186/s41232-023-00269-3

Moradi, S., Mahdizadeh, H., & Šarić, T. (2019). Research and therapy with induced pluripotent stem cells (iPSCs): Social, legal, and ethical considerations. *Stem Cell Research & Therapy, 10(341).* https://stemcellres.biomedcentral.com/articles/10.1186/s13287-019-1455-y

nmdp. (2018, September 5). *Tips for a gradual return to healthy exercise habits after transplant.* https://bethematch.org/blog/health-and-transplant/tips-for-a-gradual-return-to-healthy-exercise-habits-after-transplant/

Petersen, A., MacGregor, C., & Munsie, M. (2014, July 16). *Stem cell tourism exploits people by marketing hope.* The Conversation. https://theconversation.com/stem-cell-tourism-exploits-people-by-marketing-hope-29146

Regenerative Orthopedic Institute. (2021, August 20). *What kind of doctor is best for stem cell therapy?* https://www.regenerativeorthopedicinstitute.com/what-kind-of-doctor-is-best-for-stem-cell-therapy/

Regenesis. (n.d.). *Is stem cell therapy covered by insurance?*

https://regenesisstemcell.com/faq/will-insurance-cover-stem-cell-therapy

Riordan, N. (2017). *Stem cell therapy for chronic disease: An interview with Dr. Neil Riordan (Part 1)*. Riordan Clinic. https://riordanclinic.org/2017/09/stem-cell-therapy-chronic-disease-interview-dr-neil-riordan-part-1/

Santhosh, C. (2024, April 18). *FDA warns about stem cell therapies*. WTAQ. https://wtaq.com/2024/04/18/us-fda-mandates-label-updates-on-car-t-cancer-therapies/

Scudellari, M. (2016, June 15). How iPS cells changed the world. *Nature, 534,* 310–312. https://www.nature.com/articles/534310a

Shihadeh, H. (2015). *History and recent advances of stem cell biology and the implications for human health* [Honors project]. University of Rhode Island. https://digitalcommons.uri.edu/cgi/viewcontent.cgi?article=1432&context=srhonorsprog

Shin, J., Ryu, C., Yu, H., Shin, D., & Choo, M. (2020, February). Current and future directions of stem cell therapy for bladder dysfunction. *Stem Cell Reviews and Reports, 16(1),* 82–93. https://www.ncbi.nlm.nih.gov/pmc/articles/PMC6987049/

Shivarkar, A. (2023, July 24). *6 emerging trends in using stem cell assays*. Cell & Gene. https://www.cellandgene.com/doc/emerging-trends-in-using-stem-cell-assays-0001

Srinivasan, M., Thangaraj, S., & Ramasubramanian, K. (2021, December 1). Exploring the current trends of artificial intelligence in stem cell therapy: A systematic review. *Cureus, 13(12)*. https://www.cureus.com/articles/78128-exploring-the-current-trends-of-artificial-intelligence-in-stem-cell-therapy-a-systematic-review#!/

Stallard, J. (2023, November 10). *Disrupting a single gene could improve CAR T cell immunotherapy, new study shows*. Memorial Sloan Kettering Cancer Center. https://www.mskcc.org/news/disrupting-single-gene-could-improve-car-cell-immunotherapy-according-to-new-study

Stemedix. (n.d.). *Financing options*. https://stemedix.com/financing/

Sugarman, J. (2008). Ethical issues in stem cell research and treatment. *Cell Research 18 (Suppl 1)*, S176. https://www.nature.com/articles/cr2008266

Terashvili, M., & Bosnjak, Z. (2019, January). Stem cell therapies in cardiovascular disease. *Journal of*

Cardiothoracic and Vascular Anesthesia, 33(1), 209–222. https://www.ncbi.nlm.nih.gov/pmc/articles/PMC6203676/

Trawczynski, M., Liu, G., David, B. T., & Fessler, R. G. (2019). Restoring motor neurons in spinal cord injury with induced pluripotent stem cells. *Frontiers in Cellular Neuroscience, 13(369)*. https://www.frontiersin.org/articles/10.3389/fncel.2019.00369/full

Tucker, M. (2023, July 3). *33% of type 1 diabetes patients insulin-free with stem cells*. Medscape. https://www.medscape.com/viewarticle/993974

UCLA Health. (n.d.). *Bone marrow/stem cell transplant patient stories*. https://www.uclahealth.org/medical-services/transplants/bone-marrowstem-cell-transplant/patient-stories

UPMC. (n.d.). *Stem cell transplant diet*. https://www.upmc.com/-/media/upmc/patients-visitors/education/unique-pdfs/stemcelltransdiet.pdf

Vicsek, L., & Gergely, J. (2011). Media presentation and public understanding of stem cells and stem cell research in Hungary. *New Genetics and Society, 30(1)*, 1–26. https://www.tandfonline.com/doi/full/10.1080/14636

778.2011.552297

What are stem cells? (n.d.) University of Rochester Medical Center. https://www.urmc.rochester.edu/encyclopedia/content.aspx?contenttypeid=160&contentid=38#

Wendler, R. (2022, June 14). *Autologous stem cell transplants: What to expect.* MD Anderson Cancer Center. https://www.mdanderson.org/cancerwise/what-are-autologous-stem-cell-transplants.h00-159540534.html

West, M. (2021, August 5). *Does Medicare cover stem cell therapy?* MedicalNewsToday. https://www.medicalnewstoday.com/articles/does-medicare-cover-stem-cell-therapy

Wollert, K. & Drexler, H. (2005, February 4). Clinical applications of stem cells for the heart. *Circulation Research, 96(2)*. https://www.ahajournals.org/doi/10.1161/01.res.0000155333.69009.63

World Health Net. (2018, November 18). *Why is stem cell therapy so expensive?* https://www.worldhealth.net/news/why-stem-cell-therapy-so-expensive

Ye, L., Swingen, C., & Zhang, J. (2013, February 1). Induced pluripotent stem cells and their potential for basic and

clinical sciences. *Current Cardiology Reviews 9(1), 63–72.*
https://www.ncbi.nlm.nih.gov/pmc/articles/PMC3584308/

Zeng, C.-W. (2023). Advancing spinal cord injury treatment through stem cell therapy: A comprehensive review of cell types, challenges, and emerging technologies in regenerative medicine. *International Journal of Molecular Sciences, 24(18),* 14349. https://pubmed.ncbi.nlm.nih.gov/37762654/

Zhang, X., Cai, J., Chen, L., Yang, Q., Tian, H., Wu, J., Ji, Z., Zheng, D., Li, Z., & Chen, Y. (2022). Mapping global trends in research of stem cell therapy for COVID-19: A bibliometric analysis. *Frontiers in Public Health, 10.* https://www.frontiersin.org/journals/public-health/articles/10.3389/fpubh.2022.1016237/full

Reading Resources

Abe, K., Yamashita, T., Takizawa, S., Kuroda, S., Kinouchi, H., & Kawahara, N. (2012). Stem cell therapy for cerebral ischemia: From basic science to clinical applications. *Journal of Cerebral Blood Flow Metabolism, 32(7),* 1317–1331. doi: 10.1038/jcbfm.2011.187

Albersen, M., Weyne, E., & Bivalacqua, T. J. (2013). Stem cell therapy for erectile dysfunction: Progress and future directions. *Sex Medicine Reviews, 1(1),* 50–64. doi:

10.1002/smrj.5

Alessandrini, M., Preynat-Seauve, O., De Bruin, K., & Pepper, M. S. (2019). Stem cell therapy for neurological disorders. *South African Medical Journal, 109(8b)*, 70–77. Doi: 10.7196/SAMJ.2019.v109i8b.14009

Arshi, A., Petrigliano, F. A., Williams, R. J., & Jones, K. J. (2020). Stem cell treatment for knee articular cartilage defects and osteoarthritis. *Current Reviews in Musculoskeletal Medicine, 13(1)*, 20–27. doi: 10.1007/s12178-020-09598-z

Bian, Y., Wang, H., Zhao, X., & Weng, X. (2022). Meniscus repair: up-to-date advances in stem cell-based therapy. *Stem Cell Research & Therapy, 13(1)*, 207. doi: 10.1186/s13287-022-02863-7

Borlongan, C. (2019, May 16). Concise review: Stem cell therapy for stroke patients: Are we there yet? *Stem Cells Transactional Medicine, 8(9)*, 983–988. https://pubmed.ncbi.nlm.nih.gov/31099181/

Chang, Y. H., Wu, K. C., Harn, H. J., Lin, S. Z., & Ding, D. C. (2018). Exosomes and stem cells in degenerative disease diagnosis and therapy. *Cell Transplant, 27(3)*, 349–363. doi: 10.1177/0963689717723636

Chu, G. Y., Chen, Y. F., Chen, H. Y., Chan, M. H., Gau, C. S.,

& Weng, S. M. (2018). Stem cell therapy on skin: Mechanisms, recent advances and drug reviewing issues. *Journal of Food and Drug Analysis, 26(1)*, 14–20. doi: 10.1016/j.jfda.2017.10.004 Borlongan, C. V. (2019).

Fleiss, B., Guillot, P. V., Titomanlio, L., Baud, O., Hagberg, H., & Gressens, P. (2014). Stem cell therapy for neonatal brain injury. *Clinics in Perinatology, 41(1)*, 133–148. doi: 10.1016/j.clp.2013.09.002

Francis Crick Institute. (2023, August 30). *Researchers identify stem cells in the thymus for the first time.* https://www.crick.ac.uk/news/2023-08-30_researchers-identify-stem-cells-in-the-thymus-for-the-first-time

German Stem Cell Network. (2020, March). *Bubble Boy, Berlin Patient, and Butterfly Girl.* https://understanding-stemcells.info/Therapy/Casestudies.aspx

German Stem Cell Network. (2020). *Patient Jack Crick.* https://understanding-stemcells.info/Portals/4/Documents_PDF/03-Therapy_PDF/patients_therapy_understanding-stemcells.pdf

Hu, L., Zhao, B., & Wang, S. (2018). Stem cell therapies for cancer in China. *Human Gene Therapy, 29(2)*, 151-157.

doi: 10.1089/hum.2017.261

Irfan, A., & Ahmed, I. (2015). Could stem cell therapy be the cure in liver cirrhosis? *Journal of Clinical and Experimental Hepatology, 5(2),* 142–146. doi: 10.1016/j.jceh.2014.03.042

Israeli, J. M., Lokeshwar, S. D., Efimenko, I. V., Masterson, T. A., & Ramasamy, R. (2022). The potential of platelet-rich plasma injections and stem cell therapy for penile rejuvenation. *International Journal of Impotence Research, 34(4),* 375–382. doi: 10.1038/s41443-021-00482-z

Kim, S. U., & de Vellis, J. (2009). Stem cell-based cell therapy in neurological diseases: a review. *Journal of Neuroscience Research, 87(10),* 2183–2200. doi: 10.1002/jnr.22054

Kingery, M. T., Manjunath, A. K., Anil, U., & Strauss, E. J. (2019). Bone marrow mesenchymal stem cell therapy and related bone marrow-derived orthobiologic therapeutics. *Current Reviews in Musculoskeletal Medicine, 12(4),* 451–459. doi: 10.1007/s12178-019-09583-1

Kosaric, N., Kiwanuka, H., & Gurtner, G. C. (2019). Stem cell therapies for wound healing. *Expert Opinion on Biological Therapy, 19(6),* 575–585. doi: 10.1080/14712598.2019.1596257

LaPar, D. J., Kron, I. L., & Yang, Z. (2009). Stem cell therapy for ischemic heart disease: Where are we? *Current Opinion in Organ Transplantation, 14(1),* 79-84. doi: 10.1097/MOT.0b013e328320d2e2

Li, R., Lin, Q. X., Liang, X. Z., Liu, G. B., Tang, H., Wang, Y., Lu, S. B., & Peng, J. (2018). Stem cell therapy for treating osteonecrosis of the femoral head: From clinical applications to related basic research. *Stem Cell Research & Therapy, 9(1),* 291. doi: 10.1186/s13287-018-1018-7

Ludwig, T., Andrews, P., Barbaric, I., Zhao, T., & Mosher, J. (2023, September 12). ISSCR standards for the use of human stem cells in basic research. *Stem Cell Reports, 18(9).* https://www.cell.com/stem-cell-reports/fulltext/S2213-6711(23)00302-8

Meyfour, A., Pahlavan, S., Mirzaei, M., Krijgsveld, J., Baharvand, H., & Salekdeh, G. H. (2021). The quest of cell surface markers for stem cell therapy. *Cellular and Molecular Life Sciences, 78(2),* 469–495. doi: 10.1007/s00018-020-03602-y

Nagaishi, K., Arimura, Y., & Fujimiya, M. (2015). Stem cell therapy for inflammatory bowel disease. *Journal of Gastroenterology, 50(3),* 280–286. doi: 10.1007/s00535-015-1040-9

Qin, H., & Zhao, A. (2020). Mesenchymal stem cell therapy for acute respiratory distress syndrome: From basic to clinics. *Protein Cell, 11(10),* 707–722. doi: 10.1007/s13238-020-00738-2

Riordan, N.H. (2017). *Stem cell therapy: A rising tide: How stem cells are disrupting medicine and transforming lives.*

Shao, A., Tu, S., Lu, J., & Zhang, J. (2019). Crosstalk between stem cell and spinal cord injury: pathophysiology and treatment strategies. *Stem Cell Research & Therapy, 10(1),* 238. doi: 10.1186/s13287-019-1357-z

Siniscalco, D., Giordano, A., & Galderisi, U. (2012). Novel insights in basic and applied stem cell therapy. *Journal of Cell Physiology, 227(5),* 2283–2286. doi: 10.1002/jcp.22945

Sivan, P. P., Syed, S., Mok, P. L., Higuchi, A., Murugan, K., Alarfaj, A. A., Munusamy, M. A., Awang Hamat, R., Umezawa, A., & Kumar, S. (2016). Stem cell therapy for treatment of ocular disorders. *Stem Cells International,* 2016, 8304879. doi: 10.1155/2016/8304879

Trounson, A., Kolaja, K., Petersen, T., Weber, K., McVean, M., & Funk, K. A. (2015). Stem Cell Research. *International Journal of Toxicology, 34(4),* 349–351. doi: 10.1177/1091581815581423

Wan, X. X., Zhang, D. Y., Khan, M. A., Zheng, S. Y., Hu, X.

M., Zhang, Q., Yang, R. H., & Xiong, K. (2022). Stem cell transplantation in the treatment of Type 1 Diabetes Mellitus: From insulin replacement to beta-cell replacement. *Frontiers in Endocrinology (Lausanne), 13,* 859638. doi: 10.3389/fendo.2022.859638

Wang, X. X., Zhang, L., & Lu, Y. (2023). Advances in the molecular pathogenesis and cell therapy of stress urinary incontinence. *Frontiers in Cell & Developmental Biology, 11,* 1090386. doi: 10.3389/fcell.2023.1090386

Wertheim, J. A., & Leventhal, J. R. (2015). Clinical implications of basic science discoveries: Induced pluripotent stem cell therapy in transplantation—a potential role for immunologic tolerance. *American Journal of Transplantation, 15(4),* 88–890. doi: 10.1111/ajt.13155

Wilkinson, A. C., Ishida, R., Kikuchi, M., Sudo, K., Morita, M., Crisostomo, R. V., Yamamoto, R., Loh, K. M., Nakamura, Y., Watanabe, M., Nakauchi, H., & Yamazaki, S. (2019). Long-term ex vivo haematopoietic-stem-cell expansion allows nonconditioned transplantation. *Nature, 571(7763),* 117–121. doi: 10.1038/s41586-019-1244-x

Xu, Y., Jiang, Y., Xia, C., Wang, Y., Zhao, Z., & Li, T. (2020). Stem cell therapy for osteonecrosis of femoral head: Opportunities and challenges. *Regenerative Therapy, 15,*

295–304. doi: 10.1016/j.reth.2020.11.003

Yamaguchi, S., Yoshida, M., Horie, N., Satoh, K., Fukuda, Y., Ishizaka, S., Ogawa, K., Morofuji, Y., Hiu, T., Izumo, T., Kawakami, S., Nishida, N., & Matsuo, T. (2022). Stem cell therapy for acute/subacute ischemic stroke with a focus on intraarterial stem cell transplantation: From basic research to clinical trials. *Bioengineering (Basel), 10(1),* 33. doi: 10.3390/bioengineering10010033